Latin American Perspectives on the Sociology of Health and Illness

The sociology of health and illness is a rapidly growing field. Yet, as a field, it has suffered from a remarkably limited perspective dominated by scholarship produced in the global north. Scholars in the sociology of health and illness have been late to enter debates in global health and have generally failed to learn lessons from work originating in the global south. To begin to address this limitation, this edited collection features notable contributions from Latin American scholars exploring key issues, including sickle cell disease in Brazil, cancer and Chagas disease in Argentina and reproductive health in Mexico. This collection, offering a snapshot of the rich and nuanced research being conducted in the region, offers readers valuable lessons. It is our argument that Latin American health sociology has much to offer the larger field of sociology – both for what it can teach us about Latin America in and of itself, and for what this field of scholarship can teach us about health and illness as broadly defined. This collection challenges readers to think about the global nature of health inequalities. Rich in empirical data and theoretical substance, this book is an essential collection for readers interested in understanding the sociology of health and illness.

The chapters in this book were originally published as a special issue of *Health Sociology Review* and as individual papers in *Global Public Health* and *Critical Public Health*.

Fernando G. De Maio is Associate Professor of Sociology at DePaul University, Chicago, USA.

Ignacio Llovet is Full Professor of Sociology at Universidad Nacional de Luján, Buenos Aires, Argentina.

Graciela Dinardi is Professor of Research Methods at Universidad Nacional de Tres de Febrero, Buenos Aires, Argentina.

Latin American Perspectives on the Sociology of Health and Illness

Edited by
Fernando G. De Maio, Ignacio Llovet
and Graciela Dinardi

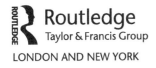

Routledge
Taylor & Francis Group

LONDON AND NEW YORK

First published 2019
by Routledge
2 Park Square, Milton Park, Abingdon, Oxon, OX14 4RN, UK

and by Routledge
52 Vanderbilt Avenue, New York, NY 10017, USA

First issued in paperback 2020

Routledge is an imprint of the Taylor & Francis Group, an informa business

© 2019 Taylor & Francis

British Library Cataloguing-in-Publication Data
A catalogue record for this book is available from the British Library

ISBN 13: 978-0-367-66416-9 (pbk)
ISBN 13: 978-0-367-00184-1 (hbk)

Typeset in Minion Pro
by codeMantra

Publisher's Note
The publisher accepts responsibility for any inconsistencies that may have arisen during the conversion of this book from journal articles to book chapters, namely the possible inclusion of journal terminology.

Disclaimer
Every effort has been made to contact copyright holders for their permission to reprint material in this book. The publishers would be grateful to hear from any copyright holder who is not here acknowledged and will undertake to rectify any errors or omissions in future editions of this book.

Contents

CONTENTS

Citation Information

The following chapters were originally published in the *Health Sociology Review*, volume 26, issue 3 (November 2017). When citing this material, please use the original page numbering for each article, as follows:

Chapter 1
Blurred logics behind frontline staff decision-making for cancer control in Argentina
Natalia Luxardo and Hernán Manzelli
Health Sociology Review, volume 26, issue 3 (November 2017) pp. 224–238

Chapter 2
Sexual and reproductive health: perceptions of indigenous migrant women in northwestern Mexico
Lourdes Camarena Ojinaga, Christine Alysse von Glascoe, Evarista Arellano García and Concepción Martínez Valdés
Health Sociology Review, volume 26, issue 3 (November 2017) pp. 239–253

Chapter 3
Reproductive health and Bolivian migration in restrictive contexts of access to the health system in Córdoba, Argentina
Lila Aizenberg and Brígida Baeza
Health Sociology Review, volume 26, issue 3 (November 2017) pp. 254–265

Chapter 4
Doctor–patient relationships amid changes in contemporary society: a view from the health communication field
Mónica Petracci, Patricia K. N. Schwarz, Victoria I. Ma. Sánchez Antelo and Ana María Mendes Diz
Health Sociology Review, volume 26, issue 3 (November 2017) pp. 266–279

Chapter 5
Social disparities producing health inequities and shaping sickle cell disorder in Brazil
Clarice Santos Mota, Karl Atkin, Leny A. Trad and Ana Luisa A. Dias
Health Sociology Review, volume 26, issue 3 (November 2017) pp. 280–292

Chapter 6

Socio/Ethno-epidemiologies: proposals and possibilities from the Latin American production
Anahi Sy
Health Sociology Review, volume 26, issue 3 (November 2017) pp. 293–307

The following chapters were originally published in *Global Public Health* and *Critical Public Health*. When citing this material, please use the original page numbering for each article, as follows:

Chapter 7

Mitigating social and health inequities: Community participation and Chagas disease in rural Argentina
Ignacio Llovet, Graciela Dinardi and Fernando G. De Maio
Global Public Health, volume 6, issue 4 (June 2011) pp. 371–384

Chapter 8

Chagas disease in non-endemic countries: 'sick immigrant' phobia or a public health concern?
Fernando G. De Maio, Ignacio Llovet and Graciela Dinardi
Critical Public Health, volume 24, issue 3 (2014) pp. 372–380

Chapter 9

Extending the income inequality hypothesis: Ecological results from the 2005 and 2009 Argentine National Risk Factor Surveys
Fernando G. De Maio, Bruno Linetzky, Daniel Ferrante and Nancy L. Fleischer
Global Public Health, volume 7, issue 6 (July 2012) pp. 635–647

For any permission-related enquiries please visit:
http://www.tandfonline.com/page/help/permissions

Notes on Contributors

Lila Aizenberg is affiliated with the National Council of Technical and Scientific Investigations in the Centre of Investigations Regarding Culture and Society at the National University of Córdoba, Argentina.

Evarista Arellano García is Professor in the Facultad de Ciencias at the Universidad Autónoma de Baja California, Ensenada, Mexico.

Karl Atkin is Head of the Department of Health Sciences at the University of York, UK.

Brígida Baeza is affiliated with the National Council of Technical and Scientific Investigations in the Institute of Social and Political Studies at the National University of Patagonia, Comodoro Rivadavia, Argentina.

Lourdes Camarena Ojinaga is based in the Facultad de Ciencias Administrativas y Sociales at the Universidad Autónoma de Baja California, Ensenada, Mexico.

Fernando G. De Maio is Associate Professor of Sociology at DePaul University, Chicago, USA.

Ana Luisa A. Dias is a Ph.D. Student in the Department of Health Sciences at the University of York, UK.

Graciela Dinardi is Professor of Research Methods at Universidad Nacional de Tres de Febrero, Buenos Aires, Argentina.

Daniel Ferrante is affiliated with the Ministerio de Salud de la Nación, Buenos Aires, Argentina.

Nancy L. Fleischer is Assistant Professor of Epidemiology in the School of Public Health at the University of Michigan, Ann Arbor, USA.

Bruno Linetzky currently works in the Medical Department at Eli Lilly, Indianapolis, USA. His research involves diabetology, epidemiology and public health.

Ignacio Llovet is Full Professor of Sociology at Universidad Nacional de Luján, Buenos Aires, Argentina.

Natalia Luxardo is a faculty member in Consejo Nacional de Investigaciones Científicas y Técnicas at the University of Buenos Aires, Argentina.

Hernán Manzelli is a Research Associate in the Centro de Estudios de Población at the University of Buenos Aires, Argentina.

Concepción Martínez Valdés is based in the Facultad de Ciencias Administrativas y Sociales at the Universidad Autónoma de Baja California, Ensenada, Mexico.

Ana María Mendes Diz is based in the Facultad de Ciencias Sociales in Consejo Nacional de Investigaciones Científicas y Técnicas at the University of Buenos Aires, Argentina.

Clarice Santos Mota is based in the Department of Collective Health at the Universidade Federal da Bahia, Salvador, Brazil.

Mónica Petracci is based in the Facultad de Ciencias Sociales at the University of Buenos Aires, Argentina.

Victoria I. Ma. Sánchez Antelo is based at both the University of Buenos Aires and Universidad Nacional de Tres de Febrero, Buenos Aires, Argentina.

Patricia K. N. Schwarz is based in the Facultad de Ciencias Sociales in Consejo Nacional de Investigaciones Científicas y Técnicas at the University of Buenos Aires, Argentina.

Anahi Sy is a Researcher in the Instituto de Salud Colectiva at Universidad Nacional de Lanús, Buenos Aires, Argentina.

Leny A. Trad is based in the Department of Collective Health at the Universidade Federal da Bahia, Salvador, Brazil.

Christine Alysse von Glascoe is based in the Departamento de Estudios de Población at El Colegio de la Frontera Norte, Tijuana, Mexico.

Introduction: Latin American perspectives on the sociology of health and illness

Fernando G. De Maio, Ignacio Llovet and Graciela Dinardi

Introduction

The sociology of health literature, for the most part, has not been global in its thinking – being late to enter debates in global health and failing to learn lessons from work in the global south (Cockerham & Cockerham, 2010; De Maio, 2014). Standard sociology of health and illness textbooks rarely take a global perspective – often relegating global health to an isolated chapter, disconnected from fundamental concepts and theories. Yet we know that global health offers important lessons for us all; indeed, a consensus may be emerging that global health should be defined not by location ("out there") but by the scope of the problem and its determinants (Koplan et al., 2009). Latin American health sociology shows the value of this approach.

It is our argument that Latin American health sociology has much to offer the larger field of sociology – both for what it can teach us about Latin America in and of itself, and for what this field of scholarship can teach us about health and illness broadly defined (De Maio, 2010). Mirroring Raewyn Connell's argument in *Southern Theory* (2007), we believe that Latin American health sociology offers us lessons that we should learn *from*, and not just learn *about*.[1]

Latin American health sociology developed under an array of historical, contextual and intellectual factors (Montagner, 2008). The field was influenced by medical anthropology, public health and medicine (among other disciplines) – with each perspective helping to shape the identification of problems, the collection of data, and the definition of research agendas. Perhaps most importantly, the Latin American tradition of *social medicine* – focused on the study of social inequality and the way in which it determines health–illness processes – influenced health sociology in the region (Barreto, 2004; Castro, 2001). This interest in the issue of social inequality has had a lasting impact on global health, which in recent decades has similarly began to acknowledge inequality as a fundamental cause of illness (without always recognizing the historical lineage of the idea).

Latin American health sociology has also been influenced by the general epidemiological profiles of countries in the region. Thus, it has been said that the region "faces typical dynamics of a modern context with the still important burden of what characterizes the old models" (Di Cesare, 2011). Earlier yet, Briceño-León (2003) had underlined that since the epidemiological transition in the region had not been completed, the sociology of health had to deal with both the new and the old epidemiological patterns. In his words, "the sociology of health in Latin America is at the same time a sociology of the living conditions of poverty and of the lifestyles of the abundance" (Briceño-León, 2003).

The region faces ongoing challenges from neglected diseases as well as pressures from chronic noncommunicable diseases, all mapping on to what Paul Farmer (2005) calls the "fault lines of inequality". These challenges coexist with an uneven progress – within and between countries – that the region has experienced in terms of access to (and quality of) health care (Lozano, 2018).

Politically and demographically, the last four decades have been remarkably complex in the region – with the rise and fall of authoritarian regimes, boom and bust economic cycles, armed conflict, large population shifts, and uneven / contested relationships in global trade. And to be sure, many of these issues remain unresolved. As we write this introduction, there are ongoing political and economic crises in Argentina, Brazil, Nicaragua and Venezuela. Latin American health sociology – with a lineage to social medicine – clearly identifies these macrolevel issues within its purview as fundamental causes of poor health.

Yet despite a rich history of scholarship, contributions from health sociologists in Latin America have not featured in recent work published in English-language journals nor in health sociology's best-selling textbooks. As a contribution to the development of this topic, this book presents a set of nine articles that examine Latin American issues and populations, six of which were previously published in a special issue of *Health Sociology Review*. In the original call for the special issue, we encouraged contributions from scholars based in Latin America, although the call was open to any scholar writing about Latin American issues or using ideas, methods and concepts of work especially oriented to Latin America. We received many notable submissions (in Spanish and English), and we are pleased to present this collection with works by authors from Argentina, Brazil and Mexico. While this collection is not (and was not meant to be) representative of the totality of the sociology of health in Latin America, we believe that these documents offer readers a valuable insight into that tradition.

Aizenberg and Baeza explore reproductive health among Bolivian migrant women in Argentina. Drawing on qualitative in-depth interviews, the authors inquired how Bolivian women living outside their home country dealt with obstacles to accessing the formal health system while remaining connected to their traditional knowledge and community networks. Luxardo and Manzelli discuss the mechanisms for priority setting for the care of cancer patients in a health-care center in Argentina. Using an ethnographic methodology, they identified different accounts that guided the decisions of practitioners. This mode of priority setting impacted the quality of health provision and reinforced mechanisms of inequality. Mota, Atkin, Trad and Dias examine social disparities and health inequalities in the context of sickle cell disorder in Brazil. They explore a chronic disease with high levels of mortality that primarily affects nonwhite populations, documenting how the lack of timely treatment in vulnerable populations impairs quality of life. The authors examine how the dual burden of social inequality and racial discrimination impacts the disease experience of those with this genetic condition.

Sy offers a theoretically and methodologically grounded proposal for the development of ethno-epidemiology and sociocultural epidemiology. This implies an approach to the field of health that the author Sy positions as an original development originating in Latin America. This development integrates the epidemiological perspective with those coming from the fields of sociology and medical anthropology. Petracci, Schwarz, Sánchez Antelo and Mendes Diz examine the patient–physician relationship from a health communications perspective. They identify three axes of the patient–physician relationship: patient satisfaction, relationship models between both and ehealth. The latter is highlighted as the main current focus of reflection and research. Von Glascoe, Arellano García and Martínez Valdés investigate the experiences of indigenous migrant women in México in their contact with health services. The article shows how during that experience sociocultural factors are brought into play and women appropriate their bodies and re-signify their sexual and reproductive rights.

Llovet, Dinardi and De Maio compare different intervention strategies for surveillance and control of a neglected disease primarily associated with poverty, and a major driver of health inequity – Chagas disease – in northern rural Argentina. They show that strategies based on community participation may be effective in reducing the social patterning of the burden of disease, even in poor places. From a more global perspective, De Maio, Llovet and Dinardi focus their interest on the process of securitization of global health and the "risk" represented by neglected tropical diseases for populations, as in the case of Chagas disease, in non-endemic countries and one of its consequences, which is to shift the attention of the poor populations of the global south to the well-to-do populations of the global north. Finally, De Maio, Linetzky, Ferrante and Fleischer test the association between income inequality and self-assessed health in Argentina for 2005 and 2009, drawing attention to the need for new theoretical models that explain how inequalities in different parts of the income spectrum can influence population health.

In bringing together these articles, we hope to stimulate thinking among health sociologists over the need for our discipline to take seriously the global nature of health and illness. Population health, as we have seen time and time again in Latin America, is socially determined by global forces, and health systems are similarly affected by transnational policies. To understand the local, we must grapple with the global, and this applies in both the global north and the global south.

References

Barreto, M. L. (2004). The globalization of epidemiology: Critical thoughts from Latin America. *International Journal of Epidemiology*, 33(5), 1132–1137.

Briceño-León, R. (2003). Endemias, epidemias y modas: la sociología de la salud en América Latina. *Revista Española de Sociología*, 3, 69–85.

Castro, R. (2001). Sociología médica en México: el último cuarto de siglo. *Revista Mexicana de Sociología*, 63(3), 271–293.

Cockerham, G., & Cockerham, W. C. (2010). *Health and globalization*. Cambridge: Polity.

Connell, R. (2007). *Southern theory: The global dynamics of knowledge in social science*. Cambridge: Polity.

Di Cesare, M. (2011). El perfil epidemiológico de América Latina y el Caribe: desafíos, límites y acciones. LC/W.395 CEPAL.

De Maio, F. G. (2010). *Health & social theory*. Basingstoke: Palgrave Macmillan.

De Maio, F. G. (2014). *Global health inequities: A sociological perspective*. Basingstoke: Palgrave Macmillan.

Farmer, P. (2005). *Pathologies of power: Health, human rights, and the new war on the poor*. Berkeley: University of California Press.

Koplan, J. P., Bond, T. C., Merson, M. H., Reddy, K. S., Rodriguez, M. H., Sewankambo, N. K., et al. (2009). Towards a common definition of global health. *Lancet*, 373(9679), 1993–1995.

Lozano, R. (2018). Measuring performance on the Healthcare Access and Quality Index for 195 countries and territories and selected subnational locations: A systematic analysis from the Global Burden of Disease Study 2016. *Lancet, 391*, 2236–2271.

Montagner, M. A. (2008). Sociologia Médica, Sociologia da Saúde ou Medicina Social? Um Escorço Comparativo entre França e Brasil. *Saúde e Sociedade (São Paulo), 17*(2), 193–210.

Note

1. Connell argues, "colonized and peripheral societies produce social thought *about the modern world* which has as much intellectual power as metropolitan social thought, and more political relevance" (2007: xii).

Blurred logics behind frontline staff decision-making for cancer control in Argentina

Natalia Luxardo and Hernán Manzelli

ABSTRACT

In this article we approach socioeconomic inequities in cancer by examining a particular dimension of health care: how health services attending patients with cancer set priorities for their daily activities. By using qualitative ethnographic data, we explore logics underlying how practitioners make priority-setting decisions regarding cancer prevention and care. We found four main types of accounts: accounts based on macro social inequalities, accounts based on patients' social and cultural features, accounts based on characteristics of health services, and accounts based on personal voluntarism. These blurred logics shape the everyday decisions which have an impact not only on the quality of health care in general but on the increasing socioeconomic inequities in cancer care attention.

Introduction

Cancer is a leading cause of death and disability in low and middle income countries (Farmer et al., 2010). Differences in the incidence, prevalence, mortality, as well as the burden of cancer exist not only among developed and developing countries but also in specific population groups within countries. People from low income strata are generally diagnosed at later stages of the disease and tend to get less therapeutic care (World Health Organization [WHO], 2008). Epidemiological studies show that these disparities occur as a result of many different factors, such as unequal access to health care, socioeconomic factors, hazardous labour and environmental conditions, nutrition and differences in health behaviours (Marmot & Wilkinson, 2006; McMullin & Weiner, 2008). Moreover, certain issues keep people from seeking prevention and care at early stages of the disease, namely lack of awareness of the importance of screening and early detection, the stigma associated with cancer, and economic barriers (WHO, 2008).

There is a broad literature on determinants of health, as well as the social structures that generate them; although most determinants of health and illness are situated outside the health care sector (Black, 1980; Bouchard, Albertini, & Batista, 2012; Marmot, 2004), some are deeply implicated in the needs and access to health care (Angus et al., 2013; Broom &

Doron, 2011; King, Chen, Dagher, Holt, & Thomas, 2014). For example, the gap between the resources of health services and the needs and expectations of different population groups, as well as significant variations in how physicians carry out diagnostic and therapeutic decisions depending on their patients' gender, age, income -among other characteristics- may contribute to inequalities in health care (King et al., 2014; Peck & Denney, 2012).

This study is anchored within literature of equity that examines the linkage between socio-economic and health care inequalities, focusing on concrete mechanisms by which specific cancer disparities are generated (Gould, 2004; Sinding & Wiernikowski, 2009). This is well documented across the continuum of cancer control – understood as the strategy to 'attack' cancer globally that includes primary prevention, early diagnosis, treatment and palliative care- for different populations (King et al., 2014; Sinding, 2010).

There is a broad spectrum of possible perspectives which can be used to analyze the inner workings of the health care sector, one of them being connected to the process of decision-making. Taking decisions and establishing priorities is a daily activity in every health care system around the world and, consequently, there is a robust, interdisciplinary field of knowledge on the issue. As Hunink et al. (2014, p. 1) mentioned 'decisions in health care can be particularly awkward, involving a complex web of diagnostic and therapeutic uncertainties, patient preferences and values, and costs'. Decision makers are the ones who are designated to make choices on different alternatives. They are responsible for aligning available resources with institutional priorities, for managing the day-to-day activities in health services and, in some cases, for producing the official guidelines of how to proceed in different scenarios. However, as previous research has found, a great deal of everyday decision-making and priority-setting occurs on the front lines, carried out by bedside physicians, administrative clerks, and other health care professionals (Baltussen & Niessen, 2006; Martin, Abelson, & Singer, 2002). In addition to the medical and economic dimensions – as well as patients' preferences and values inscribed in diverse contexts- there is a far less analyzed dimension which is that of the socio-cultural and organisational aspects which may permeate important decisions and priority-setting by health system personnel.

In a previous ethnographic study which explored some relevant features of the social treatment of cancer in Argentina's health services (Luxardo & Manzelli, 2015) we observed subtle, implicit and repeated narratives from health professionals on making decisions and establishing priority-settings in oncology services which go far beyond the guidelines included in their official programs and protocols. Routine activities in a health service require taking decisions that are not deemed 'important enough' to be included in the official guidelines or to merit seeking instructions from authorities. These were small, everyday decisions. We observed that this kind of ad-hoc decision-making and priority-setting would sometimes shape or reproduce some aspects of the social and economic inequities among patients with cancer. In general, these actions had a more negative impact on health interventions given to patients from a lower economic stratum, with a lower level of education or from specific ethnic groups (e.g. indigenous peoples). These initial findings drove us to explore in more depth the underlying logics of the daily establishment of priorities or decision-making.

What decisions were taken on a daily basis and how they were experienced by professionals in oncology health services? How were these decisions taken? Which accounts by health services' staff explained them? Were decisions consensual or, on the contrary, were they a source of friction among staff? These new, inductively derived findings directed our attention towards theoretical concepts such as decision-making and priority-setting, but as they actually take place in health services every day, rather than as they are formally depicted in official documents and programs.

In this article we distance ourselves from the classical economic models of decision-making theory usually developed in Administration, which deem decision-making to mean the rational, deliberate and purposeful actions that occur in every organisation (Tarter & Hoy, 1998). Furthermore, we avoid delving into conceptual discussions on what decision-making, priority setting or resource allocation mean for various theories and only briefly define them from the single perspective taken in this study, simply in order to specify the terms' theoretical implications.

We support a flexible, broad definition of decision-making which responds to research interests. In other words, we need to understand what happens from the point of view of our informants. The issue of how professionals participate in priority-setting is usually presented in connection with micro-level priority-setting performed by physicians at bedside, but we extend it to the rest of staff, given that they also make daily decisions on cancer care and prevention (Martin et al., 2002).

In Argentina, cancer is the second leading cause of death (Abriata, Roques, Macías, & Loria, 2012). The IARC Report (WHO, 2008) states that the region of Latin America is experiencing the greatest cancer burden, and identifies the following as the main problems in public health when dealing with cancer: having to diagnose at advanced stages of the disease, poor access and quality of cancer treatments, limited access to affordable cancer drugs, poorly trained health personnel, weak epidemiological surveillance and low priority and resources for cancer in the public health agenda.

The country has a mixed health system with three sectors: public, social security and private; they have different population coverage, services and funding. Penckaszadeh, Leone, and Rovere (2010) state that it has been an increased fragmentation, inequity and inefficacy, as health care is increasingly prey to economic interests of private corporations, trade union bureaucracies and the medical professional establishments. All provinces and the City of Buenos Aires are autonomous in implementing public health policies. The public system is underfinanced and deteriorated, with access barriers and low quality of care and one-third of the patients that receive care in the public sector have some type of social security coverage (Penckaszadeh et al., 2010).

In this article, we aim to advance our understanding of the socioeconomic inequities in cancer. A particular dimension of healthcare is examined: the process of decision-making and priority setting in daily activities in health services. More specifically, the general aim of this article is to explore and describe how health services' staffs establish priority-setting decisions on cancer prevention and cancer care interventions and the accountability or the thinking behind the staffs' decisions or priorities. To this end, we used qualitative perspectives using data proceeding from ethnographic fieldwork conducted in oncology health services in Argentina in 2012 and 2013.

Methods

This article presents the specific results of a larger project which was carried out in oncology health services throughout Argentina during the years 2012 and 2013, and was supported by the National Cancer Institute (INC). The purpose of the study was to describe the most relevant features in the social treatment of cancer, specifically in connection with the provision of health care to patients with this disease. Using an ethnographic approach, we analyzed the views of stakeholders, staff members, patients as well as their family caregivers on the different dimensions of health care provision.

The type of analysis that we follow in this article is embedded in a qualitative research tradition known as reanalysis, which is still being defined and debated (Wasterfors, Akerstrom, & Jacobson, 2014.)

Reanalysis can be described as a type of secondary analysis that relies on primary sources. It includes any second look at previously collected data picked from any source, such as archives or interviews. We also carried out a supplementary analysis based on data generated by the same research team, exploring some aspects that had previously gone unnoticed and were unexplored in the theory.

Data was taken from interviews conducted during the Primary Study (PS) period (2012–2013) with staffs of sixteen hospitals and fourteen health centres attending patients with cancer. The facilities varied in size, region and type. At least two hospitals and two health centres were included from each region of Argentina -Northwest, Northeast, *Cuyo*, Center, Patagonia and the Buenos Aires metropolitan area.

The study subjects totalled 40 health professionals (physicians, nurses, social workers and psychologists). This sample was selected purposively: professionals who (1) were currently working in any area of cancer prevention and/or cancer care; (2) belonged to different positions within the broad umbrella of roles and disciplines that are in charge of cancer control. Only professionals from the public sector were included. Thirty were interviewed by NL: seventeen physicians (specialising in Oncology, Gynecology and Clinical Medicine), eight nurses, three psychologists and two social workers. In order to obtain the same type of data from all of Argentina, we included interviews conducted by other members of the research team that also carried out the PS (Fernández, Bengochea, Durand, & Hong, 2015).

It is noticed that the main criterion for selecting the interviews for this article was the presence of the codes under our new analysis. The structure of the final theoretical sample, with 40 cases is balanced in terms of the characteristics of the interviewees (gender, position, region). The potential bias in the limitations of the study refers to those interviewees that do not accept to answer the questions, the response bias, this is a common bias for this type of study.

We utilised a semi-structured questionnaire with open questions which discussed different phases in cancer control specifically geared towards interviewees' different positions and disciplines. Most interviews were audio taped but for certain topics some respondents felt uneasy and chose not to be taped.

Different strategies for conducting interviews were implemented *in vivo* according to the context. The characteristics of the settings where we developed our fieldwork demanded being alert and sensitive to institutional contingencies that occurred during the information-gathering process.

The PS was approved by local Ethics Committees and approved by the INC. All interviews were confidential. Also, in order to prevent the possibility of interviewees being identified we did not identify provinces but rather the country's six main regions. Consent was obtained by explaining to the participating subjects our main objective and scope of the research project. We made clear that the use of collected data would not be restricted to a final report but would be shared and discussed with health services' teams and policy makers. The main goal of obtaining this data was to become better acquainted with current conditions, guiding an informed transformation of everyday activities in health services treating patients with cancer. Considering that the purpose of this reanalysis of primary data is closely related to the aims and the scope of the PS, it is understood that this query is covered by the terms under which consent was originally obtained.

In order to process and analyze the qualitative data, we followed an interpretative tradition which seeks to understand in detail the multiple, diverse positions to which social actors adhere, and locates these positions within a broader range of underlying beliefs, perspectives and/or agendas (Charmaz, 2005). This perspective takes an in-depth exploratory approach to data collection, aimed at documenting the subjective and complex experiences of the respondents.

Findings

Frontline practitioners accounts for establishing priorities

The process of setting priorities in giving care to patients with cancer is shaped mostly by the day-to-day activities at the health services frontlines. Official guidelines and program protocols play an important role in taking such decisions, but restricting these processes to written documents obscures a great part of what is going on at health services. There is an indispensable, interpretative action behind the understanding of those guidelines.

This interpretive action of understanding and implementing program guidelines and protocols is permeated by skepticism that some health workers feel about these tools (Luxardo & Manzelli, 2015). A critical distance from these tools generates a window of opportunity for individual considerations on priority-setting processes in daily activities in health services. In a heuristic effort to analyze some of the accounts on establishing priorities, we found reasoning that may have resulted in decisions that shaped some aspects of the social and economic inequities among patients with cancer.

'Better something than nothing' versus 'Better nothing than fabrications': accounts based on macro social inequalities

A key reasoning that guides health personnel when having to establish priorities is considering the structural vulnerability prevalent in the communities where each health service is located. Specifically, their target population finds itself in a vulnerable situation within society and this is something with which health services have to deal. Thus, priority-setting at the frontline is rooted in one of two logics: either a pragmatic logic that deals with what is possible given limited resources; or the gold standard logic, closer to what is clinically recommended. This is a position of context versus content: both include making decisions about types and spaces for treatment, ways of disclosing diagnoses, and referrals.

Often, the task of setting priorities is based on what resources are available, without taking into consideration other issues that fall outside the scope of the intervention. Oncologists have to decide on treatments whose supply is restricted or rather rely on obsolete therapies which are no longer recommended. This may lead them to decide to refer patients to private practices, where they can get the right kind of treatment. As one physician explained:

> We have good oncologists, good centres, professionals with excellent training, our team is first rate ... yet we are failing at specific treatments. Oncology drugs are usually covered in the Province's programs -and delivered on time- but we lack high complexity equipment for specific treatments. Radiotherapy (...) we had a cobalt bomb which is not working right now. Thus, all those type of treatments have to be paid out of pocket. (Male doctor, hospital from Central Region in Fernández et al., 2015, pp. 122–123.)

This perspective relies on an external objective reality that health services are unable to change, and this social impossibility of change is extended to health care activities, leading to a cycle of decline in already poor interventions. In this regard, the quality of practices for cancer prevention may be questionable, given the oft-repeated axiom: 'What are you going to do? At least this is better than nothing.' They suggest that, as doctors working for the public service and vulnerable populations, they must take decisions that help people gain access to 'at least' some type of care, affected by factors that constrains the quality of treatment in those settings: labour strikes, shortage of professionals, equipment for tests, treatments that do not work, waiting times for appointments running up to months, having to stand in line for hours, among others. Some professionals take into consideration contextual factors in their daily practices.

In extreme situations, and in the worst settings, cancer is just the tip of the iceberg for an entire situation of exclusion. If this tip emerges by blowing up to the surface, all other problems, whether associated or not with the disease, would require support and responses that an already frail institution could not afford. Like Pandora's Box, it is best kept closed. As one clinical doctor put it:

> Being diagnosed with cancer is the least serious thing they could have in their life. Alcoholism, unemployment, drugs, malnutrition, domestic violence, sexual abuse ... what can our institution do with all of that? (...) We choose just to leave things as they are now; let the person go back to his hovel with the problem that brought them here solved. Is this the best practice? No. It's the practice that we can afford. (Female clinical doctor from hospital in Northwest region)

In contrast, there is another perspective which sustains that health workers cannot reduce the thresholds of medical attention in the name of benefiting the poor. Thus among professionals conflicts arise that are rooted in these two confronted visions of how to make proper decisions: to consider what is clinically recommended or to consider the context and what is possible for that particular reality (the lesser of two evils).

An interesting example provided by our interviewees is about a specific program for genital and breast cancer. Gynecologists resisted the proposal, supported by many clinic and generalist practitioners at the first level (where people in rural areas go for first attention), of 'opening' certain practices, typically considered as belonging to their own specialty (e.g. taking PAP samples) to the scope of other specialists, such as clinicians or generalists. This proposal is defended by the latter as a strategy to give women the opportunity of early detection as soon as they contact the institution, considering that this may turn out to be the only chance that they have at early detection. These professionals maintain that even when certain diagnoses practices (e.g. colposcopy) should not be transferred, others -also useful for cancer prevention- very well can be.

Some professionals resist becoming an accomplice to the subtle 'vacating' of the health system, instead of demanding what are considered the best practices in clinical care. Two gynecologists referred to this situation as the proposal of 'poor medicine for the poor' and mentioned the pressures they face in this regard, considering that epidemiological surveillance relies on numbers rather than quality, so what is important is that procedures be done (no matter how). One weighty argument for this side is the huge number of mistaken diagnoses oncologists have found in the disease trajectories of people at advanced stages of cancer.

What is at stake here is to what extent quality standards must be followed -or sacrificed- in order to have, at the very least, something realistic to implement. Oncologists have their international clinical practices for treatments, however, due to the lack of resources and other factors, they sometimes decide to lower thresholds depending on what is possible. Another example of how these two perspectives influence priority-settings processes appears in the case of breast cancer. Most surgeons believe that plastic surgery should be practiced on the same day as the mastectomy. However, this is often unfeasible because of difficulties in raising the money for breast prostheses.

> I'd like to implant the breast prosthesis at the same time as the mastectomy, even when there are indications against doing so. I talked to several people and they asked 'where will you get the money for the breast prosthesis?' and so on … they only throw a spanner in the works … it's a general deterioration of the hospital … The less we do, the better.. (Male doctor, hospital from City of Buenos Aires in Fernández et al., 2015, p. 108)

As a consequence, priority-setting in treatments lays out minimum and maximum quality standards. As this oncologist doctor points out:

> First, access to brachytherapy … Do we have it? It's a good start. Second, we need to optimize the time between treatments, and try to avoid delays. If we have no brachytherapy, external beam plus boost is better than nothing. And if there is no boost, we'll only do external beam.. (Medical doctor, peri-urban Buenos Aires in Bengochea, 2015, p. 168)

The opposite situation is mentioned by oncologists who believe that the quality in medical service will determine the patient's chances to live or die. Thus, for radiotherapy, they prioritise quality over comfort so, whenever possible, they choose to refer patients to radiotherapy centres that are further from their residences but which they know to be appropriate.

These dilemmas were also mentioned with rural patients. Travel to treatment cancer services -available in urban areas- was pointed out as a subtle pressure when deciding referrals and types of treatment. Patients diagnosed with cancer living in rural areas many times insist on the need to rush to be out of home in the shortest period possible, even when they could not find neither treatment facilities nor biomedical oncological expertise at home. So, medical doctors have to deal with this when deciding.

'Taking care of themselves is just not in them': accounts based on social and cultural characteristics of the patients

Another important line of reasoning when establishing priorities is related with the social and cultural characteristics of the target population. Health service staffs have vast experience and knowledge about the population they are working with. The fact that guidelines and program protocols generally ignore this knowledge was one of the sources of the skepticism that health workers have about them. This lack of attention to cultural specificities in the guidelines leaves room for individual and personal decisions.

In interviews held in the countryside, doctors expressed that they lack interlocutors to implement preventive programs so it is nearly impossible to get one off the ground. Community referents such as nurses, teachers, administrative staff, are also immersed in very unfavourable contexts.

This reasoning acquires tangible complexity in fundamental decisions such as the diagnostic disclosure. Some medical doctors expressed that they often doubt whether to disclose cancer to their patients. They stated that all the problems associated with this disclosure would generate a worse reality, because, at any rate, patients would be unable to take action in initiating their care.

During the fieldwork we found that prejudices and stereotypes on the target population have influence on the inequality of care. These stereotypes may possibly activate a self-fulfilling prophecy, such as shorter time for consultation because they 'won't follow any medical prescription anyway'; untrustworthy relationship in the clinical encounter since 'they [patients] only come for emergencies', condescendence 'I don't lose my time giving explanations. Medical language it's hard to understand for them' and others.

Health workers will insist on and dedicate efforts to proposals that they consider fruitful in advance or, on the contrary, they will rapidly give up on projects they consider pointless. For example, in the countryside, the staff stated that the lack of education of rural workers is liable to render proper measures for cancer control futile.

> The Province's Health Ministry wanted a strategy of primary care attention that would enable rural workers to do their job while being protected against chemicals which are responsible for many types of cancer. You know, such as wearing masks when fumigating crops, the appropriate boots, so that all their clothes wouldn't be full of chemicals ... but we gave up. Taking care of themselves is just not in them. They wear the boots one day and the next day ... barefoot again. (Male nurse, hospital from Northeast region)

'The health services that we have': accounts based on characteristics of the health services

Four main aspects emerged in the intrinsic limitations of the health system: bureaucratic rules, negligence, labour conditions and political influence.

Bureaucratic mechanisms in social insurance for the poor were named as responsible for reducing physicians' potential to choose between treatments. As stated by an oncologist: 'our hands are tied' with regards to best practices, since following international guidelines is almost impossible due to insurance requisites. Access to medication or medical tests is denied. The lack of drugs in countryside institutions has been noted: 'Not even basic drugs, not to mention monoclonal antibody therapy'.

Another example of these bureaucratic obstacles is related with radiology services. Doctors said that they must complete a radiotherapy treatment in order to be authorised to schedule new appointments for the second phase of treatment. But this requisite causes delays that work against optimal timing:

> I'm not allowed to schedule a brachytherapy appointment until the patient has completed radiotherapy, which is insane ... if there are any administrative obstacles, as there usually

are, the patient might have to wait for two months … the quality of that kind of radiotherapy is the worst because the timing is wrong. (Male doctor from Central region, Bengochea, 2015, p. 169.)

The geographic location of patients is considered a central issue for therapeutic success because many treatments fail due to the times between radiology sessions. 'We ask the patient to lie and leave some information blank when filling forms on health insurance'. Having certain types of health insurance or living in certain locations may mean that patients are denied treatments, medications, or practices. In the treatment of cervical cancer, each day of delay between external radiotherapy and localised therapy reduces the chances of five-year survival. As a result, referring to a specific specialist is frequently a medical option, not a protocol to be followed.

The way health systems organise their logistics is also considered an obstacle. Taking the prevention of cervical cancer again as an example, doctors mentioned complications brought about by delays in obtaining biopsies. Extractions are taken in one place, analyzed in another and later must return to the first place of attention. The problem is with the most vulnerable population: if people never return to pick up results of their biopsies, there are no institutional mechanisms to follow up on these unclaimed tests. Patients' circumstances are outside of the scope of the institution.

Priority-setting for cancer control also includes 'partial' or even the 'absence of' making decisions. Negligence in different areas of the health system has become naturalised by some health workers. Several interviewees mentioned that issues of logistics are underestimated, which sometimes causes a loss of previous efforts made by prevention programs. For instance, staff involved in cervical cancer programs talked about the problems of biological samples obtained with PAP tests. These professionals stated that quite often samples become useless because after extraction, they were never delivered to the proper place in time to be analyzed. These interviewees recalled not uncommon episodes in which half of the glassware containing cervix samples were broken in transport. They also discussed samples that were not in proper conditions: no spray, in bad hygienic conditions and later contaminated, among others.

One important decision that frontline oncologists must take is whether to disclose to patients that have been wrongly diagnosed that their disease is at advanced stages because of inefficient attention. Blaming colleagues is not an option: most of the time these errors are obscured by blurred explanations to patients and family about why they are now in such advanced situation. Many examples were mentioned: gynecologists who do not do medical transfers on time, dentists that dismiss sore spots in the mouth, throat specialists that keep patients on antibiotic treatment after long-lasting sore throats.

Physicians dealing with high complexity believe that their colleagues of the first level of attention should not be blamed for erring diagnoses and/or treatments. As one specialist interviewed stated:

I think professionals do their best, everything they can do, but they don't have enough training. It's a matter of expertise, of specific training. Everything now is within a protocol; there are norms, guides of clinical practices. (Male oncologist from city of Buenos Aires, Fernández et al., 2015, p. 127.)

Some interviewees listed labour conditions in the public health system among the factors that affect the priority-setting process. Low salaries and poor working conditions (e.g. part-time or temporary work) result in health workers taking on multiple jobs, double shifts, private practices, outpatient care. With the pretext of their low salaries, some health centre professionals work fewer hours than scheduled, which in turn causes the health service to be particularly saturated because of the reduced consultation hours.

> They [staff] complain about labor conditions and make an 'ad hoc' act of justice for themselves by working fewer hours … but in the end, when you check the overall picture, well … it's not a bad salary for just two hours of work! (Male doctor from a health centre in the Central region.)

There is no political decision to demand that these professionals do what they are expected to do because it would mean a discussion on raising salaries. At the same time, nor is there the political will to improve job conditions. In this way, the reduction of working hours becomes naturalised as a way of maximising low salaries.

Another element influencing priority-setting processes is that of political influence. Economic and human resources are distributed among programs according to local political mileage. In this sense, cancer is a political matter. For example, some interviewees expressed that cancers affecting the blood system are disdained by hospital managers. They cannot capitalise success in these treatments because they require high investment combined with poor visibility or social recognition. Hematologists reported that at local health care practices, patients with cancer in the blood system tend to be rejected due to the complexity of these cases. Dismissing patients with this type of cancer is an unspoken policy among hospital administrators: '[this type of patient] is a problem that no one wants to deal with'.

At the other extreme, certain practices with great visibility and good reputations drain the scarce resources, mostly guided by the logic of 'showing off'. Oncologists at high complexity hospitals in the North-East region complained to us about their institutional websites sometimes offering certain medical residencies which exceed their real capacity, posted without checking with the hospital first. Programs focused on children and women receive more funding. Moreover, funds spent on visible investments and building infrastructure are lacking in other less obvious areas, such as chemotherapy chairs.

Political influence is also an important factor determining who can really take decisions. Priority setting does not always depend on a hospital's formal organisation chart. As one director mentioned, a mayor's influence may be decisive in priority-setting, depending on what happens to be on the political agenda and consequently more politically profitable. In some hospitals, the decisive pressure is exercised by labour unions, which have the power of discarding or fomenting specific proposals.

'Just with your own effort': accounts based on personal voluntarism

The last identified logic underlying the processes of establishing priorities is a special one because it shows health workers' individual efforts to improve the quality of care for patients with cancer. Many doctors try to resolve problems with their own resources that are usually insufficient to meet the many needs.

During fieldwork we registered that some health services staff take great pains to help patients, and take an active role in obtaining what is needed. They turn to personal contacts that are key to getting attention, drugs, certain type of tests, and referrals. However, the patient's case depends on the diligence of the staff member, and ultimately, on the empathy between the patient and the health service staff member. What is underlying here is a logic of doing a patient a favour which falls beyond the actual responsibilities of the job. They may, for example, help get a difficult to obtain appointment for a lab test, the proper medication for completing treatment or an authorisation from the health insurance for a referral.

Throughout all the focused ethnographies and interviews we held, we identified traits of personal logic behind institutions that impinge particular characteristics which depend on human factors, in addition to structural conditions. There are staffs that counterbalance the tight constraints in cancer care through their good will and extra efforts, as one male nurse said sarcastically: 'Whenever it works, it's because you put your heart – and I would add your blood, sweat and tears also- into it'. Reversely, as was already mentioned, there are also those who only make things worse through their negligence and lack of commitment but also their resignation, an attribute we noted in more than a few health providers' narratives, justified in the adverse context where they belong:

> You learn to be in automatic pilot ... You choose to be a clinical doctor in a rural health center because your ideals to change reality are strong. But when month after month, the only answers you get to your requests are excuses made by corrupt politicians ... and you see all your efforts go to waste, hierarchies based on political contacts and no training, well ... let me put it this way: you just throw in the towel. (Male doctor, health centre from Northwest Region)

Thus, we observed that many times referrals to specialists are made outside of protocol, based on associations between the personnel of different services, and on the level of commitment and the initiative of the staff. One social worker remarked:

> When nobody can find a way to make an appointment for a certain test in time, we go to Ana, the administrator, and beg her to change the doctor's schedule. She always finds a spot. (Female social worker, hospital from the city of Buenos Aires)

Many social workers, nurses and psychologists we interviewed mentioned that some doctors make referrals to specialists 'hanging in the air', in other words without taking into consideration the context and the feasibility of the orders requested. This omission may lead to the intervention eventually failing. This was illustrated by one nurse:

> 'The oncologist sent a patient to have radiation therapy in one place that, due to cost-cutting measures, had few professionals to do the sessions'.

Often, the desire to help patients also goes beyond their expertise. It may lead to incorrect diagnoses, and subsequently, futile treatments that only delay proper care. Clinicians at the first level try to solve health problems with what they have at their disposal. The ability to care for patients along a continuum of response or clinical outcome includes clinicians' deciding when to refer patients to other health care professionals. Doctors say their colleagues are reluctant to refer patients because it may look as if they lack the resources or technical competence to provide a response. Some doctors also indicated that health insurance institutions pressure them into not making medical referrals or requesting complex lab tests.

Finally, two main issues were found as positive within this context. One, the rewards of doing their job with dignity despite circumstances, the sense of feeling good by helping others and receiving gratitude from them and their families. The other positive side staff mentioned was the teamwork, the feeling of 'belonging' and cooperation among them was also found rewarding.

Discussion

In this article we explored the logics of health service staffs which shape priority-setting processes. We were particularly interested in narratives that would result in small, daily actions of social inequality in the attention of patients with cancer. The accounts for priority-setting were not only rationales but also contingencies for applying them, pragmatic decisions staff must make on a daily basis, and finally, the absence or uncertain decisions made or not made with no more reasons than emotional and intuitive excuses.

We identified some logics underlying the priority-setting process by describing four main types of accounts: accounts based on macro social inequalities, accounts based on the social and cultural characteristics of the patients, accounts based on the characteristics of health services, and accounts based on personal voluntarism. The findings of this article illustrate how health workers' priority-setting processes have an impact not only on the quality of health care in general but on the increasing socioeconomic inequities in health care of patients with cancer in particular by practices adopted to fit in such adverse context/population. The impact of this sort of adaptive intervention, according to the context, many times implies a deterioration of the quality of the medicine, which means in the end, getting poor medicine for the poor. Broom and Doron (2011) have studied in India how this sort of bad quality intervention reproduces inequity in cancer care. Also McMullin and Weiner (2008) speak out against these types of 'discarded care'. In the study of Sinding and Wiernikowski (2009), they quoted an oncologist who speaks about offering more conservative treatment to older people with fewer social supports.

We share the arguments of Angus et al. (2013), supporting the idea that health services and procedures can reinforce and complicate patients' economic vulnerabilities, considering that barriers, constraints, deterrents were systemic features of the health care and delivery system. For example, through obstacles for doing referrals, making appointments on time, lack of agreement with the considered unfair eligibility for coverage, constant service cutbacks, hospitals directors' reduction of the budget for not 'political profitable' interventions, the arbitrary use of public resources according to what can be much more visible, among others.

As other authors state, inequitable conditions of life, such as poverty, unemployment, class' relations, insurance status among others interact to form health inequalities at the individual-level chronic disease like cancer (Angus et al., 2013). This article shed a tiny light on how health workers' priority-setting processes have an impact not only in the quality of health care in general but in increasing the socioeconomic inequities in cancer care attention.

These findings also reveal some possible directions for policy making. Excessive reliance on official guidelines and program protocols conducts to a comfort zone for everybody involved except the patients: policy makers are doing their job by elaborating guidelines and health workers are doing their job by applying the guidelines but 'adapted' to real conditions. As Jones and colleagues remarked

The dynamics of change -generated by resource scarcity and community demands – are faster than can be accommodated by traditional strategic planning processes, which are seldom sufficiently responsive to rapidly changing environmental and operating conditions. Long-term plans are routinely pre-empted by immediate pressures and contingencies (Jones et al., 2002, p. 2).

Even when it is clear that official guidelines and program protocols are fundamental for taking decisions and establishing priorities, they need to be complemented by other mechanisms which leave room for health workers to actively participate in adapting these guidelines to real everyday situations in health services. Disregarding these interpretative actions that tend to take place when applying official guidelines leaves the door open for personal and arbitrary interpretations of the guidelines which, as we have observed, impact on socioeconomic inequities in health care for patients with cancer.

Although there have been attempts to increase the quality of care in oncology services across the country in Argentina -for example through the creation of the National Cancer Institute in 2010 and the development of specific programs for cervix, breast and colon cancer- most are still in their early stages. We think that it is a good opportunity for creating mechanisms that intensify and guide the involvement of frontline health workers through active participation and that would include the perspectives of patients and their families.

Conclusions

This research also presents some limitations. The most salient is the possible presence of a bias in the sample because some health workers refused to be interviewed. Moreover, the relatively small number of staff selected for a study at the national level may limit the scope of the results. A study with a larger sample would provide more evidence on the ways that health workers interact with patients with cancer. Another limitation is the lack of a theoretical background with which to discuss and propose models of priority-setting on the day-to-day basis. It presents issues that should be analyzed in greater depth in future research. The concept of priority-setting at health services' frontlines allow to rethink some of the daily decisions taken by health workers more critically. Another interesting topic for future analysis is go deeper in explaining how these small, daily decisions perpetuate greater socioeconomic inequality in patients with cancer.

We aim to contribute with concrete insights, operative indicators and evidence that might lead to better understanding of how decisions are taken in health services attending patients with cancer in a middle income country.

Disclosure statement

No potential conflict of interest was reported by the authors.

References

Abriata, G., Roques, L. F., Macías, G., & Loria, D. (2012). *Atlas de Mortalidad por Cáncer. Argentina 2007–2011*. Buenos Aires: Instituto Nacional del Cáncer, Ministerio de Salud.

Angus, J. E., Lombardo, A., Lowndes, R. H., Cechetto, N., Ahmad, F., & Bierman, A. S. (2013). Beyond barriers in studying disparities in women's access to health services in Ontario, Canada: A qualitative metasynthesis. *Qualitative Health Research, 23*(4), 476–494.

Baltussen, R., & Niessen, L. (2006). Priority setting of health interventions: The need for multi-criteria decision analysis. *Cost Effectiveness and Resource Allocation, 4,* 14.

Bengochea, L. (2015). Escuchando a los radioterapeutas para identificar a los desafíos venideros. In N. Luxardo & L. Bengochea (Eds.), *Cancer and society. Multiple standpoints, perspectives, focuses* (pp. 157–171). Buenos Aires: Editorial Biblos.

Black, S. D. (1980). *Inequalities in health: Report of a research working group.* Londres: Department of Health and Social Security.

Bouchard, L., Albertini, M., & Batista, R. (2012). Bibliometric study of research on health inequalities. Second ISA forum of Sociology. Distributed paper.

Broom, A., & Doron, A. (2011). The rise of cancer in urban India: Cultural understandings, structural inequalities and the emergence of the clinic. *Health: An Interdisciplinary Journal for the Social Study of Health, Illness and Medicine, 16*(3), 250–266.

Charmaz, K. (2005). Grounded theory in the 21st Century. Applications for advancing social justice studies. In N. Denzin & I. Lincoln (Eds.), *The sage handbook of qualitative research* (pp. 507–536). Thousands Oaks, London and New Delhi: SAGE Publications.

Farmer, P., Frenk, J., Knaul, F. M., Shulman, L. N., Alleyne, G., Armstrong, L., … Seffrin, J. R. (2010). Expansion of cancer care and control in countries of low and middle income: A call to action. *The Lancet, 376,* 1186–1193.

Fernández, S., Bengochea, L., Durand, A., & Hong, I. W. (2015). La perspectiva de decisores e intergrantes de los equipo de salud sobre prevención y atención. In N. Luxardo & L. Bengochea (Eds.), *Cancer and society. Multiple standpoints, perspectives, focuses* (pp. 107–156). Buenos Aires: Editorial Biblos.

Gould, J. (2004). Lower-income women with breast cancer: Interacting with cancer treatment and income security systems. *Canadian Woman Studies, 24*(1), 31–36.

Hunink, M., Weinstein, M., Wittenberg, E., Drummond, M., Pliskin, J., Wong, J., & Glasziou, P. (2014). *Decision making in health and medicine integrating evidence and values* (2nd ed.). Cambridge: Cambridge University Press.

Jones, C., Keresztes, C., Macdonald, K., Martin, D., Singer, P., & Walker, H. (2002). *Priority-setting in Ontario's hospitals: Management report.* Canada: Queen's Center for Health Services and Policy Research. The Joint Center for Bioethics, University of Toronto, The Change Foundation.

King, C. J., Chen, J., Dagher, R. K., Holt, C. L., & Thomas, S. B. (2014). Decomposing differences in medical care access among cancer survivors by race and ethnicity. *American Journal of Medical Quality, 30,* 1–11.

Luxardo, N., & Manzelli, H. (2015). Clinical narratives: Cancer attention from providers and patients. In N. Luxardo & L. Bengochea (Eds.), *Cancer and Society. Multiple standpoints, perspectives, focuses* (pp. 319–386). Buenos Aires: Editorial Biblos.

Marmot, M. (2004). *Status syndrome.* Londres: Blumsbury.

Marmot, M., & Wilkinson, R. (Eds.). (2006). *Social determinants of health* (2nd ed.). Oxford: Oxford University Press.

Martin, D., Abelson, J., & Singer, P. (2002). Participation in health care priority-setting through the eyes of the participants. *Journal of Health Services Research & Policy, 7*(4), 222–229.

McMullin, J., & Weiner, D. (2008). Introduction: An anthropology of cancer. In J. McMullin & D. Weiner (Eds.), *Confronting cancer: Metaphors, advocacy and anthropology* (pp. 30–27). Santa Fe: School of Advanced Research Press.

Peck, M., & Denney, M. (2012). Disparities in the conduct of the medical encounter: The effects of physician and patient race and gender. *SAGE Open, 2,* 1–14.

Penckaszadeh, V. B., Leone, F., & Rovere, M. (2010). The health system in Argentina: An unequal struggle between equity and the market. *Italian Journal of Public Health, 7*(4), 350–358.

Sinding, C. (2010). Using institutional ethnography to understand the production of health care disparities. *Qualitative Health Research, 20*(12), 1656–1663.

Sinding, C., & Wiernikowski, J. (2009). Treatment decision making and its discontents. *Social Work in Health Care*, 48(6), 614–634.

Tarter, C. J., & Hoy, W. K. (1998). Toward a contingency theory of decision making. *Journal of Educational Administration*, 36(3), 212–228.

Wasterfors, D., Akerstrom, M., & Jacobson, K. (2014). Reanalysis of qualitative data. In F. Uwe (Ed.), *the sage handbook of qualitative data analysis* (pp. 467–480). Los Angeles and London: Sage.

World Health Organization. (2008). *World cancer report 2008*. Edited by P. Boyle and B. Lewin. Lyon: International Agency for Research on Cancer/WHO.

Note

All the verbatims that are presented in this article originated in interviews carried out during the research for *Cancer Morbidity and Mortality in Argentina, Interdisciplinary Study on the Diagnostic, Therapeutic Paths and End of Life of People with Cancer Diseases*, funded by the National Cancer Institute of Argentina. Some of the interviews were made by the authors of this article. In this case, the verbatims that are presented are considered as primary sources. Other verbatims were extracted from previous publications of other authors, for their re-analysis. They are cited as secondary sources, e.g. author, publication year and page number.

Sexual and reproductive health: perceptions of indigenous migrant women in northwestern Mexico

Lourdes Camarena Ojinaga, Christine Alysse von Glascoe, Evarista Arellano García and Concepción Martínez Valdés

ABSTRACT

This article presents a preliminary view of perceptions of the sexual and reproductive health of indigenous migrant women in an agricultural valley in Northwestern Mexico. A qualitative design was implemented with individual interviews and participatory workshops. The objective was to learn about indigenous migrant women's experiences with health services and their understanding of their sexual and reproductive rights. It was found that family was not a sufficient source of sexual information or education; that for women participating in this study, talking about sexual and reproductive health meant talking about reproduction; that the education system participates little in this aspect and that the health sector fails to respond in a timely and sufficient manner to this segment of the population. It is necessary to develop a more comprehensive view of the socio-cultural components of sexual and reproductive health in order to carry out a medical practice that considers the needs and perceptions of indigenous women. For women themselves, the challenge is to appropriate their body, to re-signify their sexual and reproductive rights and to exercise these rights.

Introduction

This article presents results of a broader investigation concerning the perceptions of sexual and reproductive health of indigenous migrant women living and working in the San Quintín valley, one of the two main agricultural valleys of northern Baja California, Mexico. This research aimed to learn about the perceptions that these women have regarding their own body, the stages of female growth and development, knowledge concerning family planning methods, traditional approaches to menstrual discomfort, care during pregnancy and puerperium, as well as their understanding of sexual and reproductive rights. Their experiences with the health services, as well as their understanding of some aspects of their sexual and reproductive health are discussed.

Over the past forty years the San Quintín Valley has become come to be an important agricultural exporter to the US market and a major centre of attraction for migrant *jornaleros* (day labourers). The intensification of commercial agriculture traditionally required a migrant workforce. The latter came from South-East Mexico, mainly from Oaxaca, Guerrero, and Veracruz, with *mixteca*, *triqui*, *zapoteca* and *nahua* ethnicities. Initially, the migration of agricultural workers was of a more temporary nature and gradually there has been a process of permanent settlement (Zlolniski, 2010). The proportion of women *jornaleras* in relation to men has increased in agricultural work because, as Lara-Flores (1995) points out, there has been a process of feminisation of agricultural labour, mainly because the female workforce is cheaper, and seen to be more docile and flexible.

Most of the studies carried out in the San Quintín area have documented that, in agricultural work, both men and women face a life of extreme poverty and working conditions below the minimum established by law, particularly if they are indigenous migrants (Lara-Flores, 2003, 2008; Velasco, 2007; Velasco, Zlolniski, & Coubes, 2014). The migrant families of the San Quintín valley live under precarious economic circumstances, specifically regarding the conditions of their homes and access to medical care. Their houses are often unsafe since some are built with waste material, without concrete flooring, with little or no ventilation and do not have basic public services (PDH-BC, 2003). Over half (57%) of the total population lacks medical attention or health services, and nearly one-third (29%) of the population 15 years of age and over, have not completed primary school studies (PDR, 2011).

In this region, most of the female migrant population has at some point in their lives worked in the agricultural fields. Some of them engage in activities such as the sale of embroidery and food as an alternative source of income. Women of early-to-advanced ages join the agricultural work force. In the case of pregnant women, they often work until the last trimester of their pregnancy. Younger girls combine agricultural labour with employment in shops or with their high school studies. Their status as women imposes additional tasks on them such as getting home after work to perform household chores and childcare. Thus, they are subjected to a double shift of paid work outside the home in addition to unpaid labour within the home. The living and working conditions of indigenous women do not allow them to have greater opportunities for well-being, and this has affected, among other things, their health. Furthermore, they have little access to health services and social security benefits, and the medical care they receive can be discriminatory and fail to meet their needs.

In addition to the marginalised nature of their lives, indigenous women also face a monocultural health care system, particularly regarding sexual and reproductive health. This gives rise to a professional indifference and disinterest in recognising women's own knowledge about their health. Regarding this, Langer and Tolbert (1998) point out that both the community and individuals should be able to have the necessary information to guarantee their freedom of choice in accordance with their cultural beliefs and practices, and have access to health and education services that protect cultural integrity. Without these conditions, this segment of the population is deprived of being able to fully exercise their sexual and reproductive rights.

The field of sexual and reproductive health continues to change, and is subject to the various interpretations of different kinds of actors. In the 90s, sexual and reproductive health became an issue of importance in the agendas of international organisations concerned with development and population policies, such as the World Conferences organised by the United Nations, and in particular the conference on Population and Development (Cairo, 1994), the Fourth World Conference on Women (Beijing, 1995), and the World Conference on Social Development (Copenhagen, 1995).

The International Conference on Population and Development (CIPD), sponsored by the United Nations took place in Cairo in 1994, and represents an event of great relevance. In this conference, new demographic paradigms were set in place that focused attention on human rights and in covering the needs of men and women. The prevailing vision previous to these international conferences regarding women's health gravitated around maternal-child health (Frenk, Gómez-Dantés, & Langer, 2012; Galoviche, 2016). The latter was replaced at the headquarters of the CIPD for a broader vision that includes sexual and reproductive health. Importantly, reproductive rights were also recognised as human rights. Galoviche (2016) points out that this position emerges from feminist struggles and gender studies, and he goes on to cite Careaga and Sierra (2006), who argued that:

> ... concerned by population growth in Third World countries, the international organisations were influenced by the strength of the global feminist movement, since they had to acknowledge that people's sexual and reproductive behaviour occurs in the context of great inequalities, among others, those of gender. (p. 165)

There were advances at Cairo's International Summit regarding sexual and reproductive health as a population issue, but also as a matter of gender. The existing power asymmetries between men and women, as well as between these institutions were also acknowledged. Thus, the CIPD outlined as its main objectives:

> ... regarding the issue of equality, equity and potentiation of the role of women, we ask governments that they guarantee the promotion and protection of women's human rights; that they sign, ratify and apply the convention on the elimination of all forms of discrimination against women and that they integrate a gender perspective in all the processes of formulation, and application of policies in the delivery of services, especially those of sexual and reproductive health. (Galdos, 2013, p. 458)

The Fourth World Conference on Women (Beijing, 1995) introduced a gender perspective into public policy as an effective way of extending this vision towards women in all aspects of their lives, including family, work and as an obligation of the State. Visualising reproductive processes and sexuality from a gender perspective highlights the historical condition of women's subordination based on unequal power over the control of their bodies, thereby sustaining their condition of vulnerability and inequality, and as subjects of violence and injustice regarding their human rights (García, 2015).

In 1995 the UN defined reproductive health as 'a complete state of physical, mental and social well-being and not only the absence of disease or suffering, in all that is relevant to the reproductive system and its functions and processes' (United Nations, 1995). Discussions at international meetings focused mainly on how to articulate different understandings of the notion of reproductive health, taking into account the interests of different actors. As Corrêa points out:

> On the one hand, the notion was developed in institutional apparatuses, sectors linked to the international system of family planning and, especially, the World Health Organization (WHO). On the other hand, similar efforts were made within women's movements; that is, the notion that reproductive health was also in the political agenda of civil societies. (2002, p. 130)

The WHO stressed the importance of both men and women exercising their sexuality autonomously and freely, as well as deciding about the number and spacing of pregnancies, complete information on contraception and access to timely care (Pedraza & Pedraza, 2014). This international health organisation conceptualised sexual and reproductive health as:

> … a state of physical, mental and social well-being in relation with sexuality. It requires a positive and respectful approach to sexuality and of sexual relations, as well as the possibility of having pleasant and safe sexual experiences, free of coercion, discrimination and violence. For sexual health to be reached and maintained, the sexual rights of all people must be respected, protected and realized. (WHO, 2002)

As a result of these reinterpretations, basic documents were developed for the elaboration of recommendations and programs targeting women, thus opening one of the most fertile fields for the application of women's rights as a fundamental part of human rights. The debate on sexual and reproductive health requires consideration of a different set of concepts such as sexual and reproductive rights, which are intertwined with fundamental human rights (Corrêa, 2001; Salles & Tuiran, 2001). According to Ortiz, the proposal that sexual and reproductive rights be conceived as human rights, is based on the universal nature of human rights that each State is obligated to ensure on behalf of its citizens, thereby making their recognition less a sign of modernity than of the State's obligation to society. Therefore, it is individuals and their rights who are able to guide the rule of law and ensure compliance (Ortiz, 1999, p. 35).

Sexual and reproductive health needs must be based on human rights, which would make it possible to take autonomous decisions and assume responsibilities both individually and collectively. These rights must be guaranteed by the State through the exercise of public policies in addition to fostering the conditions for access to health services. According to Figueroa, the exercise of reproductive rights will be feasible when social, political, legal, economic, and cultural contexts favour access to these possibilities (1999).

Cervantes points out that, between the 1960s and 1990s in Mexico, reproductive decisions went from being a private issue to being a public and government concern (1999). Health services became more oriented toward family planning with the goal of population reduction. This macro vision of women's health impeded the view of women as subjects with rights. Additionally, the existence of strong religious influences and the exclusion of women's views in the formulation of population policies hindered the full exercising of reproductive rights (Ortiz, 1999). In the last 20 years, public administration has implemented programs to respond to the commitments made at these international conferences on development and population. One of these programs, called 'Even Start in Life', was implemented in 2001, with the aim of reducing maternal mortality and morbidity-mortality in children under five years of age. In the field of sexual and reproductive health, the policy of family planning was revised incorporating new methods of planning such as the morning-after pill, the female condom and the subdermal implant. At the same time, a gender perspective was adopted that was based on two main lines of action: combating female cancer and promoting initiatives aimed at a life without violence for women. Hence, in 2006, the Mexican government enacted the *Ley General de Acceso de las Mujeres a una Vida Libre sin Violencia* (General Law on Women's Access to a Free Life Without Violence) and established the *Centro Nacional para la Equidad de Género y la Salud Reproductiva* (National Centre for Gender Equity and Reproductive Health), whose purpose is to suggest public policies related to sexual and reproductive health, and monitor and evaluate these policies, as well as the quality of health services (Frenk et al., 2012).

Mexican public policies on sexual and reproductive health have been gradually modified to better suit women. However, as García points out, these changes have occurred more in discourse than in action since 'in day-to-day life, women continue to be the main object of control, both in institutional implementation and in all [...] social relations based on the social imaginary of domesticity' (2015, p. 99). In line with this argument Salles and Tuirán point out that 'sexuality and human reproduction are embedded in structures and networks of social relations, for example, class and gender asymmetries [and ethnicity] ... Reproductive, sexual, and health care behaviours can be understood as socially structured behaviours endowed with meaning' (Salles & Tuiran, 2001, p. 99). Sexual and reproductive practices of indigenous populations are influenced by socioeconomic, educational, health, and gender inequalities, as well as the cultural nuances related to ethnic difference. Sexual and reproductive health must be thought of as a fabric of several interlocking factors where subjectivity can also be incorporated, for example, in how women live their sexuality in their daily lives, in their relationship with their partners and in their interaction with other women. This article highlights how women in this study perceive their sexuality based on their own experiences and practices.

Methodological aspects

The research was based on a qualitative design, with the participation of a total of 60 indigenous women labourers who were migrants from the southern region of the country, mainly from the state of Oaxaca, and who lived in the four different localities of the San Quintín Valley. Participants were recruited using the snowball technique. Their age range was between 17 and 60 years old in which three age groups were identified: 17–29, 30–44, and 45–60. The objective of this classification was to identify whether, in addition to intergenerational change, the migration process influenced their perceptions and practices in relation to sexual and reproductive health.

Most women over 40 years of age migrated from their place of origin at a younger age, many with their nuclear family. The younger women were born in the San Quintín region. In the latter group, half spoke an indigenous language in addition to Spanish and half did not speak their native language. Of the women who spoke their indigenous language, roughly one-third spoke *mixteco* (indigenous language from the region of Oaxaca). Regarding education, over two-thirds had either no schooling (37%) or had primary schooling only (38%); 13% had a secondary education, 10% completed high school and 2% had a bachelor's degree. Concerning current occupation, roughly half (55%) stayed at home, and the other half either worked as *jornaleras* (agricultural labourers) (23%), or were students (23%); 10% had regular employment.

Women who met the following criteria were invited to participate: identified as indigenous, spoke Spanish, had a minimum of one year residence in the locality and voluntarily consented to participate by signing a letter stating the purposes of the study and the confidentiality of the information. Two techniques were used in the field work conducted in each of the localities: participative workshops and individual interviews. Two workshops and ten interviews were carried out, which were recorded, transcribed and their content analysed. Individual interviews gathered in-depth information on the topics raised in the workshops.

The first workshop sought to obtain information on how women in the study perceived the different aspects of their sexual and reproductive health. The second explored their knowledge of the right to sexual and reproductive health, their perception of care in health services, doctor-patient interaction and how sexual health is a right for everybody. The attempt here was to determine whether these women perceived access to quality health care as their right, especially regarding sexual health.

Medical staff of the IV Health Jurisdiction of the Baja California Institute of Public Health Services, located in the San Quintín Valley, were also interviewed. It was deemed important to obtain the point of view of health services providers regarding the sexual and reproductive health and health-seeking behaviour of the indigenous female population settled in this Valley. The two nurses responsible for the Maternal Health and Female Cancer programs were interviewed, along with the doctor responsible for Family Planning and Sexual Health in Adolescents, as well as the psychologist in charge of the Violence and Gender Equity program.

Results

Sexual and reproductive health involves both biological and sociocultural processes such as the interaction of personal experiences, relationships between people, and interaction with health service providers. It also involves the broader structural context, including gender and other social and economic inequalities, sociocultural norms and practices, lack of access to education, limited employment opportunities, poor living conditions and ethnic origin, as well as political context. Results are organised under the following sub-themes: source of women's information about sexuality; onset of sexual activity and use of contraceptive methods; knowledge of sexually transmitted diseases; access to health services and doctor-patient interaction; and the exercise of sexual rights.

Source of women's information about sexuality

In the study group, women stated that their mothers did not provide sexual education such as information about the onset of menarche. Participants mentioned learning about such things from schoolmates or older sisters, information that tended to be more about personal hygiene and less about the physiological or anatomical basis of sexual development. As one interviewee commented:

> … never spoke to us about sexuality nor the changes, I have another sister that, when I started menstruating, she was the one who taught me how to put the pad because I even did not know how to put it … my sister, the middle one, started to explain–because she was the

> one with me at the time–, she told me you will put the pad, this is going to happen, but don't be afraid. (Interviewee A: 30 years of age)

In addition, talking about the intimate parts of a woman's body is very uncomfortable for older women, as shown in the following quote:

> No, we did not touch that subject because … for them, it was like disrespecting us to ask those things … did not teach me any of that, because, there, we could not talk about that, for example … of our parts or so because, for them, it was rude … (Interviewee B: 44 years of age)

Only women under the age of 40 reported having received information at school, although many felt that this information was insufficient. They commented that some teachers were reluctant or uncomfortable when teaching 'sex education'. Younger women acknowledged the importance of talking with their daughters about sexuality, although some admitted they dared not because they did not know how to approach the subject, or how to get close to their daughters. One of the youngest informants commented: 'I was told in primary school [about] what is menstruation and some parts of your body' (Interviewee C: 18 years old).

Beginning of sexual activity and contraceptive methods

In this group of women the first pregnancy often occurred between 15 and 20 years of age and the average number of pregnancies was between two and three. The following quote describes how the occurrence of pregnancies before the age of 15 years was seen as problematic: ' … yes, it is very upsetting to have 13 years old girls who are already pregnant, […] they already give all that information at school […] but what is lacking is that their parents give them some direction' (Interviewee D: 41 years old). Another interviewee pointed out: 'I did not know how to give the right information to my daughter, I did not know how to guide her, she got pregnant at age 14' (Interviewee E: 35 years old).

Participants described two types of care in pregnancy and postpartum, those provided by the health sector and traditional home care and remedies. Births tend to be vaginal rather than by caesarean section. It was common for women to carry out their prenatal care at local clinics and most births took place in local health centres, although some elected to use midwives.

Regarding family planning, most women were familiar with contraceptive methods recommended by the health sector, such as hormonal approaches and intrauterine devices. Nevertheless, not all women used a contraceptive method, whether by their own or by their partner's decision. Among those who did use them, female contraception methods were the most common. In some cases, couples discussed family planning with each other, but sociocultural barriers prevented them from communicating about sexuality with their children.

The health sector is a major source of information about sexual and reproductive health although not about sexuality or gender. One of our participants described her experience regarding information received from the health sector as follows:

> … When they tell you about sexual and reproductive health, they talk about the contraceptive methods, of when you have to go to a pap smear screening, or, for example, check your breasts for breast cancer. But the topics they do not touch, for example, are what it is to be a woman … gender difference, how do men develop … the woman … but they do not provide much information … on gender. (Interviewee F: 36 years old)

Knowledge of sexually transmitted diseases

Women are aware of the importance of screening for cervical and breast cancers, as well as for the most common sexually transmitted diseases. Not only was screening commonly available, but women showed a greater willingness to take responsibility for their health care. One of the nurses in charge of the Women's Cancer Program said that ' … I have seen advances in the indigenous population, that they are more empowered now to seek screening tests. They now make that decision'.

Access to health services and doctor-patient interaction

Concerning the use and access to health services, women often visited the health centre for general consultation, vaccine application and to carry out tests for early detection of cancer. However, basic medicines were often lacking or were insufficient. Moreover, there were no specialists available and medical equipment was often lacking. Regarding these issues, the doctor in charge of the Adolescent Reproductive Health Program mentioned:

> If we compare ourselves with Canada, if we compare ourselves with other countries that have their attention focused on health and education, the percentage of Gross Domestic Product (GDP) [of Mexico] is minimal compared to those countries (…) that also leads to different material and human resources in the area of health. And that is not the fault of the worker, nor the citizens, these are matters of political approach to health (…) the country focuses more on cure and has forgotten about the preventive side.

The health insurance program for workers provided by the Mexican National Social Security Institute provides clinics that are better equipped and where there is less rotation of medical staff. However, participants complained about the complexity of bureaucratic procedures required to access services at these clinics. Although a large proportion of women attended to their health in government-provided clinics, they also continued to use traditional medicine to treat certain diseases.

Study participants described two different types of experiences with doctors, one in which the doctor was attentive, responsible and respectful, and another where they felt discriminated against and mistreated due to their indigeneity. Figure 1 presents some of the ways participants exemplified the kinds of doctor-patient interactions they had experienced. For responsible and respectful treatment, there were phrases such as 'there are doctors who responsibly listen to people'; in contrast with discriminatory and unequal treatment, where participants said 'we wish that doctors (would) change their way of being' or 'there are doctors who make fun of their patients' health'.

Top set of notes from left to right (Figure 1):

> "we would be happy if the doctors would change the way they treat us.", "there are doctors who don't want to treat indigenous people", "we need an indigenous doctor". Second row, from left to right: "we want a female doctor who treats all people equally", "there are doctors who are responsibly listen to people". Third row, left to right: "there are doctors who understand the situation of their patients and help them", "some doctors meet their professional responsibilities, while others do not". Fourth row, from left to right: "there are doctors who do not pay attention to their patients", "there are doctors who mock their patients when they know that they should not do that". Fifth row, from left to right:

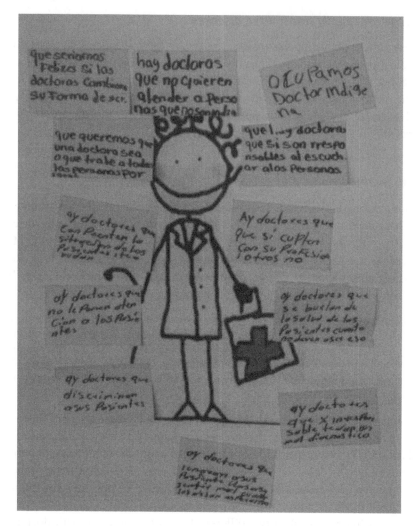

Figure 1. Perceptions of medical treatment and performance.

"there are doctors who discriminate against their patients", "there are irresponsible doctors who give you a wrong diagnosis". Sixth row: "there are doctors who ignore their patients and make us feel badly".

The training received by the health professional was often technical, and did not always provide the kinds of communication skills required for addressing issues of sexuality with adolescents, especially with indigenous populations. Relating to this issue, the doctor responsible for the Adolescent Reproductive Health and Family Planning programs mentioned that:

I did not come out [of training] sensitized [to] do Pap smears and breast cancer detections nor, much less [to] talk about family planning. I was not sensitized to that and then it is difficult for me as the head of adolescent reproductive health and family planning to sensitize medical staff (…) there is no academic training where they tell us and insist that it is very important because [in this way] violence is prevented, cancer, unplanned pregnancies, and many other things are prevented, with the simple fact of addressing sexuality at the right moment (…) we are shy talking about everything that is related to sexuality when it is necessary. Thus, as health personnel it is difficult for us to address issues of sexuality with the patients.

These omissions and deficiencies in the health sector make it more difficult for women to go to health centres and receive not only information on sexual and reproductive issues but comprehensive health care. Regarding this matter, Castro (2011) points out that when women go to health centres seeking attention on matters regarding reproductive health, the interaction with medical staff is often depersonalising, reducing the ability of women to claim their own reproductive rights. From a human rights perspective, these deficiencies constitute violations of sexual and reproductive rights.

Exercise of sexual rights

In both workshops and interviews, scarce information was obtained on how women perceive their own sexuality and whether they see themselves and their sexual partners as active agents in terms of sexual pleasure and satisfaction. Participants revealed even less about their understandings of their rights to reciprocity in their sexual relationships, that would allow them to address their own sexual needs and desires and to exercise greater control over their intimate life. One of the few interviewees who discussed her sexual rights was 24 years of age and with more schooling than most; she stated:

> … sometimes I tell him I do not want [to engage in sexual relations], and no, I want to rest, I feel tired, and sometimes, truly, he gets upset, but I tell him that I don't want to, and he has to respect me … (Interviewee G).

In one of the exercises during the workshops, some women said: 'I have the right to take care of my body and no one can force me', 'I have the right to be accepted as I am' (Figures 2 and 3). In Figure 2 the central circles says:

'I have the right to:' Around it, there are eight circles with notes in them. Moving clockwise: 'I have the right to have children to educate them, look after them and dress them', 'I decide if I work or take a break [from working]'; 'I have the right to be free and to develop myself more every day', 'I have the right to consent to sexual relations with my partner, or not'; 'I have the right to be respected by other people', 'I have the right to be respected physically and mentally'; 'I have the right to learn what rights I have', 'I have the right to decide what I want and do not want in my future'; 'I have the right to express my opinion about a topic or something important' … ; 'I have the right to insist on my rights as a person', 'I have the right to receive good treatment at work and be respected'; 'As a mother, I have the right to be respected by my children', 'I have the right to study and to express myself', 'I have the right to be respected the way I am'; 'I have the right to go out, be free, and behave myself', 'I have the right to take care of my body and no one can force me', 'I have the right to plan how many children I have or want'.

Discussion and conclusions

The impact that the education and health sectors have had in this population regarding the prevention of pregnancy is scant. This study has found that women have their first pregnancy in adolescence, some even as young as 13 years old. This coincides with the results

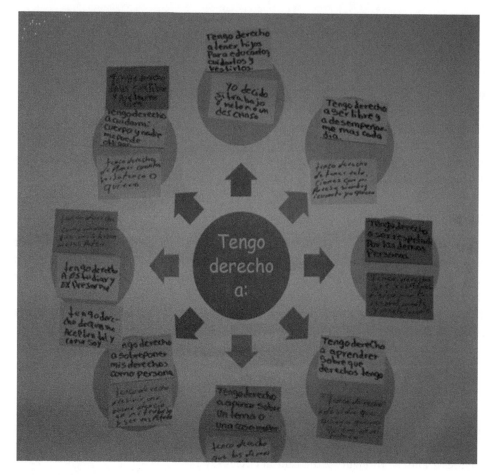

Figure 2. Poster made by the interviewees on how they perceive their rights.

published in the 2014 *Encuesta Nacional de la Dinámica Demográfica-ENADID* (National Demographic Dynamics Survey-NDDS), which shows that the average age of the first coupling of indigenous women of fertile age is within the 15–49 years of age range, almost two years younger than women who do not speak an indigenous language (INEGI, 2016).

The discourse of this group of women focuses more on reproduction than on sexuality. This makes sense when placed in the context of the health services providers' discourse, which emphasises family planning, sexually transmitted diseases and the timely detection of cervical and breast cancer, while omitting issues associated with sexuality. To talk about sexuality is, for many women, a taboo (Marston, 2004), unless it is associated with motherhood.

For a small group of these women, sexual and reproductive health implies respecting and caring for one's own body as well as being able to express emotions and to value oneself. They consider that people should be free to sustain a sexual relationship under conditions of their own choice, as well as to control their own fertility and protect

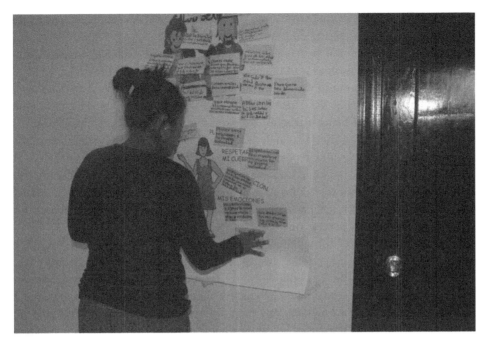

Figure 3. Poster showing one of the women adding her comment on how she perceives her sexual rights.

themselves from sexual violence. However, they do not have a specific notion of their sexual rights, since they barely recognise as such the right to bodily integrity and privacy.

For the participants of this study, the meaning of being a woman has undergone changes that can be explained by the migratory experience from rural to urban centres, and the interaction with other women. Aizenberg (2014) points out that it is the interaction between members of a community that allows the construction of social-capital bonds within the community. Migration processes expose women to a new life environment that reshapes their practices and knowledge about their sexuality. The indigenous women participating in this study who had migrated, had reconstructed their identity in constant interaction with other indigenous and non-indigenous people in this region, in daily life, in community ties, and in new jobs where they had transformed and re-signified their beliefs and perceptions.

These changes are more noticeable among younger women than older women for whom cultural norms are strongly internalised and inhibit changes in how they perceive their sexuality. Changes in life conditions are reflected in how they wish to live their sexuality and also in the way they conceive their ethnic and gender identity as subjects of law. Changes in the perception of indigenous women have meant that they not only perceive themselves as caretakers of others and are placed last among the family, but now recognise themselves as sexual beings and, therefore, begin to appropriate their body and themselves. However, the desire to live their sexuality where they can control their own fertility and protect themselves from sexual violence is not reflected in the relationships of most of the women. According to Beasley (2008), the way to increase women's ability to negotiate with their partners their intimate relationship is through sexual education, which can play an important role in preventing domestic violence.

According to the cultural beliefs of these participants, 'respectable' women do not discuss sexuality. This coincides with the findings of Karver, Sorhaindo, Wilson, and Contreras (2016), who point out in their study on indigenous women in Oaxaca, that feelings of shame and fear influence the expression of these women's sexuality. They also found that the key attribute of being a woman is linked to motherhood. Women's knowledge about their right to express their sexual desire (i.e. sexual pleasure and corporal sensuality) did not arise at the workshops reported in the Karver et al. research. Nevertheless, the current study found that for some women, the inability or unwillingness to discuss sexuality can become modified after leaving their places of origin and settling in a different environment. Interaction with indigenous and non-indigenous women about these matters can change their perceptions.

Women's perception of the quality of health care may be, among other things, an obstacle to the use of health services. Health services are focused on the medical aspects of reproduction and sexuality, as opposed to the full expression of sexuality and the promotion of the exercise of sexual and reproductive rights. Health care provided women by institutional services is not only deficient, but conforms to a unilateral institutional view that leaves aside women's needs and voices. Furthermore, indigenous women are often not treated with respect, are guaranteed neither privacy nor confidentiality and do not always receive full explanations about available services. This situation inhibits the exchange of information and encourages authoritarian treatment of doctors and other health agents towards women. It also deepens inequality in access to health services, accentuates differences and generates discrimination and social injustice.

From a social perspective, health care must focus on reducing inequalities, which in turn depends largely on the distribution of power between political actors and the role of the state, which must guarantee the exercise of health as a human right. It is therefore necessary and desirable for the health sector to have a more comprehensive view of the sociocultural components of sexual and reproductive health, so as to be able to carry out medical care in ways that takes account of the needs of indigenous women (Rodriguez-Vargas & Molina-Berrio, 2015). For this reason, it would be good to institute a series of training strategies with the goal of sensitising institutional staff on the subject of gender perspective, to aid in the promotion of access to information and guidance on sexual and reproductive health, especially for indigenous women and girls.

The full exercise of sexual and reproductive rights requires that women's partners recognise their female partner's right to decide about their own body. Here men must assume responsibility towards women's sexual and reproductive rights, which runs contrary to the traditional cultural role of men where they are permitted satisfaction of their sexual needs but have no responsibility in terms of reproduction.

The findings of the present study show that the challenge faced by health care and other institutions is to bring about changes in sexual and reproductive health care that account for the voices and needs of indigenous women. This includes not only the health sector, but also the education sector, since its role is key in sexual education, especially in the basic and higher education of the adolescent indigenous population. For women themselves the challenge is to re-establish their sexual and reproductive rights and exercise them.

More than 20 years after the International Conference on Population and Development in 1994, the need to adopt a rights perspective to approach sexual and reproductive health is still evident. This requires more than a biomedical approach to sexual and reproductive health. It is important to take into account the complex political, economic, cultural and social contexts that disadvantage broad sectors of the population such as indigenous women. To conceive and implement sexual and reproductive health from a technical standpoint is to leave aside issues of social justice.

Disclosure statement

No potential conflict of interest was reported by the authors.

Funding

This project was funded by the Comision Nacional para el Desarrollo de los Pueblos Indigenas; Comisión para el Desarrollo de los Pueblos Indígenas en México (Commission for the Development of Indigenous People in Mexico).

References

Aizenberg, L. (2014). Facilitating indigenous women's community participation in healthcare: A critical review from the social capital theory. *Health Sociology Review*, *23*(2), 91–101.

Beasley, C. (2008). The challenge of pleasure: Re-imagining sexuality and sexual health. *Health Sociology Review*, *17*(2), 151–163.

Castro, R. (2011). Teoría social y salud. In *Salud Colectiva*. Lugar Editorial, S.A., Buenos Aires.

Careaga, G., & Sierra, S. C. (2006). *Debates sobre masculinidades: poder, desarrollo, políticas públicas y ciudadanía*. México: UNAM.

Cervantes, A. (1999). Políticas de población, control de la fecundidad y derechos reproductivos: Una propuesta analítica. In B. García (Coord.), *Mujer, género y población en México* (pp. 363–429). México: COLMEX. SOMEDE.

Corrêa, S. (2001). Salud reproductiva, género y sexualidad: Legitimación y nuevas interrogantes. In C. Stern y G. Figueroa (Eds.), *Sexualidad y salud reproductiva. Avances y retos para la investigación* (pp. 127–153). México: COLMEX.

Figueroa, J. (1999). Derechos reproductivos y el espacio de las instituciones de salud: algunos apuntes sobre la experiencia mexicana. In A. Ortiz-Ortega (Comp.), *Derechos reproductivos de las mujeres: Un debate sobre justicia social en México* (pp. 147–190). México: EDAMEX.

Frenk, J., Gómez-Dantés, O., & Langer, A. (2012). A comprehensive approach to women's health: Lessons from the Mexican health reform. *BMC Women's Health*, *12*(42), 1–7.

Galdos, S. (2013). La conferencia de El Cairo y la afirmación de los derechos sexuales y reproductivos, como base para la salud sexual y reproductiva. Revista *Peruana de Medicina Experimental y Salud Pública* [online], July 30. Retrieved December 6, 2016, from http://www.redalyc.org/articulo.oa?id=36329476014

Galoviche, V. (2016). Conferencia sobre población y desarrollo de El Cairo (1994). *RevIISE*, *8*(8), 89–97.

García, M. I. (2015). El control del crecimiento de la población y las mujeres en México: organismos internacionales, sociedad civil y políticas públicas. *Revista Colombiana de Sociología*, *38*(2), 93–111.

INEGI "ESTADÍSTICAS A PROPÓSITO DEL … DÍA DE LA MADRE (10 DE MAYO)" DATOS NACIONALES. 06 DE MAYO DE 2016. Retrieved November 2, 2016, from http://www.inegi.org.mx/saladeprensa/aproposito/2016/madre2016_0.pdf

Karver, T. S., Sorhaindo, A., Wilson, K. S., & Contreras, X. (2016). Exploring intergenerational changes in perceptions of gender roles and sexuality among indigenous women in Oaxaca. *Culture, Health & Sexuality, 18*(8), 845–859.

Langer, A. y Tolbert, K. (Eds.). (1998). *Mujer: sexualidad y salud reproductiva en México*. México: EDAMEX, The Population Council.

Lara-Flores, S. (2003). Violencia y contrapoder: una ventana al mundo de las mujeres indígenas migrantes, en México. *Revista Estudios Feministas, 11*(2), 381–397.

Lara-Flores, S. (2008). ¿Es posible hablar de un trabajo decente en la agricultura moderna-empresarial en México? *El Cotidiano, 23*(147), 25–33.

Lara-Flores, S. (1995). Las empacadoras de hortalizas en Sinaloa: historia de una calificación escatimada. In A. González, & V. Salles (Coord.), *Relaciones de género y transformaciones agrarias* (pp. 165–186). México: PIEM-COLMEX.

Marston, C. (2004). Gendered communication among young people in Mexico: Implications for sexual health interventions. *Social Science & Medicine, 59*(3), 445–456. doi:10.1016/j.socscimed.2003.11.007

Ortiz, A. (Comp.). (1999). *Los derechos reproductivos de las mujeres. Un debate sobre justicia social en México*. México: EDAMEX.

PDH-BC (Procuraduría de Derechos Humanos del estado de Baja California). (2003). *Recomendación 6/2003*. Mexico: Procuraduría de Derechos Humanos del estado de Baja California.

PDR (Programa de Desarrollo Regional: San Quintin). (2011). http://imipens.org/IMIP_files/PDR-SanQuintin.pdf (Consulted July 19, 2012).

Pedraza, V. y Pedraza, I. (2014). Derecho a la salud sexual y reproductiva desde un enfoque de derechos humanos. *EN LETRA*, número extraordinario Derecho de la Salud, pp. 28–56.

Rodríguez-Vargas, F., & Molina-Berrio, D. (2015). Elementos del contexto que intervienen en el desarrollo de las políticas públicas de salud sexual y salud reproductiva elaboradas entre el 2003 y el 2013. *Revista Gerencia y Políticas de Salud, 14*(28), 10–30.

Salles, V. y Tuiran, R. (2001). Sexualidad y salud reproductiva. Avances y retos para la investigación. In C. Stern y G. Figueroa (Eds.), *Sexualidad y salud reproductiva. Avances y retos para la investigación* (pp. 93–113). México: COLMEX.

United Nations. (1995). *International conference on population and development, Cairo 5–13 September, 1994. Programme of action*, New York: United Nations, Department for Economic and Social Information and Policy Analysis.

Velasco, L. (2007). Diferenciación étnica en el Valle de San Quintín: Cambios recientes en el proceso de asentamiento y trabajo agrícola. (Un primer acercamiento a los resultados de investigación). In M. Ortega, P. Castañeda, & J. Sariego (Eds.), *Los jornaleros agrícolas, invisibles productores de riqueza* (pp. 57–78). México: Plaza y Valdés.

Velasco, L., Zlolniski, C. y Coubes, M.-L. (2014). *De Jornaleros a Colonos: Residencia, trabajo e identidad en el Valle de San Quintín*. México: COLEF.

World Health Organisation (WHO). (2002). *Sexual health*. Retrieved June 10, 2016, from www.who.int/reproductive-health/gender/sexualhealth.html#2

Zlolniski, C. (2010). Economic globalization and changing capital-labor relations in baja California's fresh-produce industry. In *The Anthropology of Labor Unions* (pp. 157–188). University Press of Colorado.

Reproductive health and Bolivian migration in restrictive contexts of access to the health system in Córdoba, Argentina

Lila Aizenberg and Brígida Baeza

ABSTRACT

Although issues of health have been thoroughly analysed in the field of migration studies, there are still very few studies that seek to understand the reproductive health of women in migratory processes. This article analyses the reproductive health of Bolivian migrant women living in the city of Córdoba, Argentina, through an analysis focused on the community assets that migrants deploy in the health-disease-care process within restrictive contexts of access to the health system. The research consisted of an exploratory study using in-depth interviews with Bolivian migrant women and health professionals through the implementation of semi-structured guidelines. The work shows that, in an environment characterised by a health system that acts to exclude, migrant women develop a series of rational strategies where they draw on community assets embodied in forms of self-care of the body and in community networks. Based on a process of reframing memories related to health practices in the Andean world, these women incorporate these assets and more easily confront the obstacles that they must overcome as migrants in different stages of their reproductive health.

Introduction

Although the understanding of the relationship between health and migration has increased in the academic literature since the mid-1980s, there is still limited understanding of the relationship regarding migration and reproductive health globally and, especially, in the Latin American region. The knowledge about the impact of migration on the health of Latin American migrant women of reproductive age, and on how the latter experience health and the care of their bodies in migratory contexts, is still scarce. Currently, the issue of reproductive health and migration deserves particular attention given the high degree of feminisation that characterises the Latin American migrant population, the high proportion of migrant women who are of reproductive age, and the challenge for the health services of the host countries to adequately address their health problems (Aizenberg, Rodríguez, & Carbonetti, 2015; Cerrutti, 2011). This article aims to fill the existing gaps in the Latin American literature from the perspective of Bolivian female migrants, coming mostly from the rural sector, and health providers that have contact with them in their host cities.

Latin America was the first region in the developing world to reach parity in the number of male and female migrants (Martínez Pizarro, 2003). Currently, of the almost 30 million people living outside their country of birth in the region, almost half are women, which represents a significant change: from predominantly men migrating at the beginning of the twentieth century, towards a gender balance in the early twenty-first century (Martínez Pizarro, Cano, & Soffia, 2014). Variations in migration flows are related to the degree of complementarity between the labour markets in the countries, labour demand in service activities, the effects of social networks and the modalities of family reunification (Martínez Pizarro et al., 2014). This international migration in Latin America has contributed to highlighting how feminisation is a salient feature of migratory processes, yet the literature has not analysed in depth the effects of migration on women's health. Until the 1990s, migrant women's experiences were invisible because analyses were often carried out from an associational perspective, women were understood as passive actors who accompanied men, which left analyses women's experiences in the migratory processes as a secondary consideration (Ariza, 2002). Nevertheless, the increasing participation of women in migration processes, the growing tendency to incorporate gender approaches in the social sciences and the conceptual opening to the figure of the migrant woman (Oso, 1998), have shown that migration processes are social phenomena shaped considerably by gender relations (Pessar & Mahler, 2003). Furthermore, in the last few years, social sciences have highlighted the need to approach the dynamic intersection between the different components present in the historical structures of domination (Lugones, 2008; Stolke, 2004). Social science analyses have demonstrated the value of the intersectionality of gender dimensions, ethnicity, social class and national origin in migration studies (Donato, Gabaccia, Holdaway, Manalasan, & Pessar, 2006), and the outcomes of the interactions (Cole, 2009) of the categories which, in the case of female migrants are placed in the social periphery. This has led to a growing attention to the relationships between migration, intra-family dynamic, the social contexts of women, impacts of displacement on gender roles and migration outcomes on the quality of life of women, including their sexual and reproductive health (Mora, 2002).

UN studies in Latin America have shown that, compared to their native counterparts, migrant women experience a higher number of unwanted pregnancies, report lower use of contraceptives and a lower propensity to attend reproductive health services (UNFPA, 2006, p. 24). In Argentina, different comparative studies (Cerrutti, 2011; INDEC, 2013) show that the average amount of prenatal care for Bolivian puerperal women is lower than for Argentine women, and that six out of ten Bolivian women have unwanted pregnancies, a situation that reveals the unmet demand for family planning services. In this sense, migration has been identified as a risk factor, showing that the confluence of gender, ethnicity, nationality and the lack of official citizenship documents can lead to the most extreme human rights violations, including sexual abuse, deterioration of reproductive health and threats to physical integrity (Martinez Pizarro & y Reboiras Finardi, 2010). Thus far, the academic approaches developed in Argentina have emphasised the different barriers that Latin American migrant women face in reproductive health. These include considerable vulnerability and exposure to diseases from living conditions in their new homes (Goldberg, 2014); the difficulties associated with access to and use of health systems (Aizenberg et al., 2015; Cerrutti, 2011); the multiple cultural processes involved with care practices and communication with the health personnel (Baeza, 2014; Jelin, Grimson, & Zamberlin, 2006), and the processes of recognition and denial of legal rights (Caggiano, 2008).

Understanding how Bolivian migrant women experience their reproductive health in Cordoba, Argentina, is of particular relevance considering the particularities of migration today. Although the presence of migrants from neighbouring countries in Argentina has always been between two and three percent of the population, in the last decades this has changed (INDEC, 2010). Currently, migration from Latin American countries to Argentina consist primarily of people born in Bolivia, Paraguay, Chile and Peru who came to Argentina as a consequence of the disadvantageous economic conditions in their countries, and the work opportunities and other favourable circumstances established in Argentina since 1990 (Cerrutti, 2011). The crisis in economies in the region and the urbanisation that has taken place has led to a decrease in the number of migrants settling in the border areas and an increase in migrants living in large urban centres, such as Cordoba. According to the 2008 provincial census, Bolivian migration is concentrated in the province's capital and the *Gran Córdoba* area and it represents 51% of the total population from bordering countries. The Bolivian people in Cordoba have typically occupied precarious and informal jobs, available in labour niches. Bolivian women tend to work in horticulture, floriculture or brick making jobs in rural or peri-urban areas, while others work in care, domestic service, textiles or sale-related activities at markets in urban areas.

In Argentina, studies have shown that South American migrants living in the country are exposed to high levels of vulnerability, bad living conditions and limited access to health services. The vast majority of South American migrants in Argentina are characterised by low levels of education, unfavourable housing conditions and scarce access to basic infrastructure services, which negatively influence their health and that of their families (Pantelides & Moreno, 2009). Furthermore, many migrants are at risk of serious diseases as result of extremely precarious working conditions or working in hazardous environments (Goldberg, 2014). In the specific case of women, migrants are even more exposed to encountering obstacles to health care services. In addition to the difficulties they have as migrants, women face obstacles due to factors associated with their social class, gender, and ethnic-cultural background (Cerrutti, 2011; Jelin et al., 2006). Thus far, those studies that have analysed the role of culture in the health of migrant women, have highlighted how cultural differences between migrant populations and the health system have generated relationships based on distrust amongst professionals and users, lack of access to modern health systems by migrant populations, low performance in women's health care, and difficulty to exercise their right to health, etc (Aizenberg et al., 2015; Baeza, 2014; Goldberg, 2014).

This article aims to analyse the way in which Bolivian migrant women in Cordoba experience the care of their reproductive health in a context of multiple barriers to the health system, favouring an analysis focused on the community assets that women deploy in the migratory experience. It is based on the conceptual assumption that Bolivian women are active agents who develop strategies and build preventive health care practices using cultural knowledge and practices that they bring from their places of origin. Particular features of the Andean culture are at play here, based in reciprocity between members of the community

(Michaux, 2004) and concepts of health and disease that are natural and holistic, which help women to navigate the different obstacles they face. Thus, this work does not seek to focus on the barriers that Bolivian migrant women must face, but rather it seeks to place women within their broader contexts where they navigate their pathways through the health-disease-care process. The literature on migration and health has focused predominantly on identifying the different obstacles that influence the access and health care of migrant women (Aizenberg et al., 2015; Baeza, 2014; Caggiano, 2008; Goldberg, 2014), without paying enough attention to how they manage to develop strategies to overcome such barriers and look after their bodies. This work incorporates a new look at the field of migration and health in Argentina, highlighting the importance of taking the migration process as an opportunity to redefine the identities of women and describe their assets as a way of coping with the difficulties encountered in the health-disease-care in their places of destination. The paper incorporates the concept of social agency as a key axis, which conceives of women as social agents and privileges their roles in, and capacities in reproducing and transmitting cultural knowledge and community networks as sources of mutual support for their health care (Anthias, 2006). In contexts of mobilities, memories are activated, certain components of the memory regarding how to care for the body in pregnancy or delivery are forcibly forgotten or silenced. Migrant women are not alone, in an intersubjective way, they are linked to families, country men and women, neighbours with whom they share experiences and affections. It is in these relationships where the practice of telling histories, news, memories concerning what was left behind in the territory of origin, where time and space overlap in a complex and dynamic way, takes place. Trigo (2011) argues that the spatial materialisation of memories becomes necessary in contexts of listening or sharing. It is in the 'lands of memory' where migrant women find the information and generationally transmitted knowledge that allows them to self-care during the pregnancy process, delivery and puerperium (Trigo, 2011, p. 11).

Focusing the study on community assets departs from the biologist approach of health as a process isolated from the social world (Good, 2003). It also departs from the neoclassic perspective of migration as an exclusively individual process (Borjas, 1989). In other words, looking at strategies that women deploy seeks to analyse the health-disease-care of migrants from a historical perspective where continuity and the resignification that Bolivian women give to traditional knowledge and practices play a key role. In this sense, this work recovers the multiplicity of spaces where women experience the bond with their bodies and their health care which are not only focused on the interpersonal relationships with doctors but located in a variety of individual and collective circumstances, recovering the explanations of the social, cultural or political causes behind the health, disease and care processes (Menéndez, 1985).

Methodological approach

The research consisted of an exploratory and descriptive study that relied on a qualitative methodology, combining in-depth interviews carried out predominantly in one of the suburbs with a large Bolivian population in the capital of Cordoba, situated in the city's periphery. Six Bolivian women were interviewed. Half of the sample were women from rural regions of La Paz and Potosí. The remaining three were women from urban centres from La Paz and Cochabamba, and members of the Andean community in

Cordoba involved in the cause of migrant rights. At the time of the interview, four women were of reproductive age (one in the 20–25 years old range, and three in the 25–35 range), had an average of two-to-three children and were users of maternal-child health services of the city's public health centres. While these migrants defined themselves primarily as Bolivians, they consider themselves in relation to their *quechua* or *aymara* ethnic origin. Seven health professionals were also interviewed (2 female doctors, 3 social workers, and 2 gynaecologist-obstetricians) working at the health centres in that suburb and general hospitals in the city of Cordoba. The information presented here is part of the field work carried out between June 2013 and December 2016. In interviews with women, the goal was to describe their trajectories and experiences with respect to their health care, especially regarding their reproductive health, as well as in specific situations such as pregnancy and childbirth. Interviews with health personnel gathered their perceptions regarding migrant populations in general, and the Bolivian flow in particular, as well as the existing barriers and facilitators in the access to and use of reproductive health services by migrant women. Although the narratives of health personnel was not exempt from the representations of the biomedical model to which they belong, in all cases they were staff who were involved in the neighbourhoods where the migrant population were based, and they carried out health practices from a perspective that reflects the trajectories of women and their needs. The project did not have the backing of any ethics committee because the funding organism did not require it. Interviewees were informed of the purpose of the interview and the voluntary nature of their participation, as well as the anonymity of the information they provided. The interviews were conducted by social researchers belonging to the university, who were presented as external and independent from health institutions. Participants were recruited through the 'snow-ball' technique. In the case of health professionals, interviews were carried out in the health services, and in the case of migrant women, in their own homes. All were recorded with consent from the interviewee and then transcribed for later processing and analysis.

Results

Although the health processes of each participants were narrativised as personal decisions of each social actors and their specific circumstances, the focus on community assets allowed the analysis of health not as an isolated 'fact' but as an historical-spatial continuity between the community to which it belongs, the country of origin and destination. The historical perspective has not been sufficiently problematised in studies of migration and health, which in their vast majority have taken migrants' stories using a static view, once they are settled in their host nation, isolating them from broader historical-social processes where they have shaped their practices and representations around their health. The historical approach invites us to take the characteristics of the health-disease-care process in the places of origin as an essential guide to highlight the diverse practices assumed by migrant groups in their places of destination. In all societies, forms of care are based on conceptions and knowledge that underlie the intervention of suffering. As Menéndez (2009) points out, the economic, political, religious, ethnic and scientific-technological development conditions that characterise a given society constitute the framework in which the different possibilities of care develop and exist. He also highlights that, even when we think of an antagonistic vision among health systems, there is a tendency, at the level of practices, to complement each other with differ-ent knowledges and forms of care, the choice of which is based on the presumptive diag-nosis made by people, as of the objective conditions that go through them.

Hence, the health and disease phenomenon occurs under a codified frame of reference, giving rise to practices and behaviours that are based on myths, ingrained believes and customs, as well as obstacles and facilitators that the subjects find along the way. As an interviewee pointed out:

> Bolivian women, have less accessibility to go to a hospital, take their children and move else-where to attend a second level of care … then they seek alternatives to follow up and there is a lot of self-care of the body that they bring from Bolivia when they don't access a (health) system … They are more careful and worried about their health and the baby inside them than Argentine (women) … more mindful of their body. There are health care and preventive attitudes by Bolivian women that Argentines do not have. In the case of breast feeding, for example, almost one-hundred percent exclusively breast feed, which Argentines do not. They have other type of habits: the majority do not smoke, do not drink alcohol during preg-nancy, in that sense, [Bolivian women] have healthier attitudes than Argentine women … (Julieta, Doctor, interview conducted in Cordoba, 7/2015).

This account points out the way in which self-care operates in the therapeutic itineraries of Bolivian migrant women as a way to counter the barriers to access the health system. According to Menéndez, self-care includes the actions developed by individuals to prevent the development of certain conditions and to favour certain aspects of health that aim to reduce risk behaviours, being the domestic group where the actions of detec-tion, diagnosis, care and healing activities of the disease are initiated (Menéndez, 2009).

The indigenous communities maintain their own perceptions of health, disease, pre-vention and healing of the individual and collective health. For many of those commu-nities, health is understood as the result of harmonious relationships with oneself, family, community and nature, which result from compliance with norms of social behav-iour and respect for the forces of nature and the elements that compose it (OPS, 2003). Within this system and as a product of the socialization and gender division, women assume the role of carer, mainly care that have to do with daily life, food and healthy body, as a symbol of the feminine figure in harmony with nature (Álvarez, Moncada, Arias, Rojas, & Contreras, 2007, p. 681). Likewise, women have played a key role as gen-erators and reproducers of social networks, carriers and transmitters of collective memory, of knowledge and culture, including the use of traditional medicine. In the interstices of the medical domain and in the face of generating greater possibilities to bring together the 'abandoned' and new territories, migrant women strongly assume the shelter of memory. By telling family histories, linking both territories through consultations, ques-tions, returns, comings and goings, memories are activated in the construction of a complex plot where the intention is to recover everything that can help to cope with the transit of migration, but in a context in which it is necessary at times to also hide, silence and in other cases forget (Baeza, 2014). These connections between the territory of origin and the new territory, as opposed to generating ruptures generate a series of approaches, contacts and new territorial ties that strengthen links and can generate new ways of knowledge transfer regarding the self-care of the body.

Thus, women resort to diverse practices for their own care, which allows them to learn their own experience, initiate themselves in the empirical knowledge in its habitat and provide self-care, a practice that they carry out to maintain their own life, health and well-being based on the knowledge they possess (Álvarez et al., 2007, p. 681).

> In Bolivia there is a very strong recognition of natural medicine and for nature, and we resort to medicinal plants that are natural to heal us because it is from earth where we are born and we heal … in the *Pachamama* (mother earth) … we believe that earth is not an object but a subject. Hence, *Pachamama* is a living being, we treat her as our mother, therefore, maternity and what arises from it, we live it as part of that nature and everything starts from that basis (Jacinta, Bolivian, interview conducted in Cordoba, 7/2015).

In this narrative, it is possible to observe the way in which the Andean worldview is reconstituted within the framework of urban life, as a way of addressing the health problems that arise in a migratory context.

These alternatives are also acknowledged by some medical professionals as valid for healing, who refer to the healing effects of plants, ointments and other elements that are part of the Andean perspectives of health. In this sense, an interviewed physician stated:

> We see here the topic of *fajar* (wrapping) the child to tighten the chest, and we ask ourselves, why? How do they look after the infant's health when they do not access the system? And we saw that the (children's) thorax was tightened with a rigid cloth because the problem (fever) was in the belly and was so that (the fever) did not go up, or the subject of urine when the child has fever, you must bath them with the mother's urine … (Julieta, Doctor, interview conducted in Cordoba, 6/2015).

The notion that self-care is an expression of the link between individual-nature health offers interesting explanations to account for the reasons underlying women's decisions when using, or not, the health system during pregnancy. In particular, the notion of self-care and understandings of pregnancy 'as something natural, as part of life', allows us to look at women's practices as resulting not only from their living conditions but as part of rational decisions, in this case based on understandings of health that go beyond the merely biological:

> Argentine (women) are more careless in many ways during pregnancy, the risk factors to which they are exposed are many. They are less respectful of their own health and that of the baby. Bolivian (women) are much more careful, naturalize the pregnancy more than an Argentine woman. (The latter) feels that pregnancy is a pathological situation, but for Bolivians pregnancy is natural, is part of life. (Carolina, Doctor, interview conducted in Cordoba, 7/2015).

Looking at migrant reproductive health from a social-historical perspective shows the dynamic-collective process that underlies women's health trajectories and allows us to account for women's ability to generate strategies according to how they interpret the context they live in and respond to it.

These situations refer to the way in which women construct their identities in line with the social fabric in which they exist, and where they bring interculturality to their various practices (Rivera Cusicanqui, 2010). As mothers, merchants, cooks, ritualists, and referents, participants health practices were built through by the similar practices that come from their place of origin and the learnings that arose from their new contexts.

> We saw and learned that there is a lot of resistance to our medical practices that had to do with a different conception of health and illness, a different healing process, and I noticed that it makes it very normal for people not to reach the health service … it is not due to

negligence but I saw that the explanations regarding disease had nothing to do with the bio-logical but with matters regarding the wind, the abandonment, the bad of the community … (Ana, social worker, interview conducted in Cordoba 9/2015).

The previous interview shows how the decision to use health services during pregnancy was based in a conscious reflection regarding women's own conception of the body and health, more than a deviation of values, obstacles or 'negligence', as it could be interpreted from the view of some health professionals. As we pointed out, the works that have addressed culture in the Bolivian migrant populations tended to look at it from the deficits that it generates. Nevertheless, as Ann Swidler points out, culture influences the actions of individuals because it provides the individual with tools, a vocabulary of meanings, symbols and repertories with which they organise their practices (Swidler, 1986).

As per Swidler (1986) we can consider the previously presented accounts to show how culture, which has usually been read as an obstacle, can be understood as part of the delib-erate strategies that women rationally implement. Far from being barriers, traditional knowledge such as self-care, are facilitators to overcome the barriers faced as migrants in the health field. Two participants offered eloquent narratives in this sense, explaining how their health problems were addressed through knowledge and practices common to the Andean worldview, despite the difficulties they encountered in health services:

> We go when we cannot do anything here anymore […] When (regarding their children) they have a stomach ache we give them a herb that is called *manzanilla* (chamomile), which we bring from Bolivia, we have good herbs, there is a tree over there for all those pains, like euca-lyptus, that is what we use. And if [the child] already has fever we bath them with eucalyptus, we boil the eucalyptus and with that water we wash their body. And also with urine, in Bolivia when you live in the country side, urine is very good for us. If it is a boy (the one with fever), it must be female urine and if it is a woman (the one with fever), boy's urine, and for the babies the urine must be from their mother and we rub it with a piece of cloth. We also put potatoes and we moist it with water and potato, we cover (the body) with that … We go to the health centre when we do not have the herbs but we only use the herbs we bring … (Roxana, Boli-vian woman, interview conducted in Cordoba, 12/2015).

> […] I don't like going (to the hospital) […] they start at 8:30 (am) but you have to wake up at 5 or 6 in the morning to take a number and you won't have an appointment until 12:30 or 1 (pm) and then you have no time to do things at home … And in the morning I have to take the children to school and every day I wait for my children, then, when they get out of school I cook or I go and pick them up … When they have fever I make them urinate. If my boy gets sick I urinate or bath him in urine, if it is my daughter I make her father urinate and rub it all over her body. If the temperature does not go down, I put ice over the head and [if the fever does not come down] well, we must go to the [health centre] (Mariela, Bolivian woman, interview conducted in Cordoba, 12/2016).

These testimonies show us how pain relief in the sick body is first sought using the knowl-edge passed through generations where the meaning acquired by the body is fundamental to think not only of the illness but the cure. The remedy comes from the body, and in this way, they intertwine with each other, oriented towards the healing.

Drawing on views of health in these cultural terms also allows us to understand that individual health is produced by historical processes that take place in a framework of social ties with characteristics specific to the migratory processes. Addressing Bolivian reproductive health from this perspective requires a closer look at the characteristics of the Bolivian migration flow in Argentina. Although Bolivian women have always been involved in the migratory processes towards Argentina, their relocation occurred within a context of family migration, unlike, for example, Peruvian women who have usually migrated alone (Magliano, Perissinotti, & Zenklusen, 2014). In migration to Argentina, the family and social networks of Bolivian migrants assume characteristics continuity and reinforcement reflecting the social bonds in the country of origin. According to Michaux, the social structure in the Andean Bolivian context is made up of 'family relations, intra-family economic and political relations, and intra-community relations that correspond to particular structures of reciprocity' (Michaux, 2004, p. 109).

The following testimony shows how the community value embedded in the system of reciprocity is part of the migrants' everyday life:

> Here there is an Andean cultural value within Bolivian collective, it is the value of the community in general ... In my family, for example, cultural diffusion is an obligation because we understand ourselves as a community, not as individuals, and that is a very [important] value. So, we must help each other because one of our inclusive values is reciprocity ... you help because at some point in life the other will help you, or you will need the other. (Noemi, Bolivian woman, interview conducted in Cordoba, 10, 2014).

This reciprocity system is fundamental for gaining access to and satisfactory transit through the health care system. As pointed out by one of the interviewees, families who had been in Argentina for longer became the "ones in charge" of transferring the information to new arrivals, including information about the health services available and the places providing the best quality care:

> The families that have been here for many years have the obligation of telling those who just arrived not only the migratory process but also where to access care ... Thus, it is for that reason that the families that have been here longer, give the information to the new ones. (Jenny, Bolivian woman, interview conducted in Cordoba, 4/2014).

The following accounts show how this reciprocity system allows women access to a support network that helps to develop care behaviours during pregnancy and childbirth, as well as information about how to overcome the geographical and economic obstacles that are present during prenatal care.

> It is very different when a Bolivian woman that has been here for a long time arrives, you see all her family outside, in the corridors waiting for the birth. They bring *mate* (traditional South American tea) and blankets to her, they help her with the baby. It is a family moment that help the woman to recover from childbirth ... the family can better support the baby and look after the mother. (Gabriela, social worker, interview conducted in Cordoba, 6/2013).

Incorporating a view that forefronts the cultural value of health for migrant Bolivian women allows us to understand that health is a historical and collective process in which the web of social bonds that are deployed become particularly relevant in the strategies that women generate. Once again, reconfiguring culture as an obstacle rather than a barrier permits a view of women's agency and their capabilities as active agents within the community contexts they live.

Here health trajectories are not analysed from the perspective of the individual but from the way women reshape the social structures and meanings present in their Andean culture and take advantage of reciprocal ties as a way to achieve a more satisfactory outcome in the sometimes hostile scenario present during specific moments of their reproductive health, such as pregnancy, childbirth and puerperium.

Conclusions

This paper aimed to observe the way in which Bolivian migrant women in Cordoba, Argentina, experienced their reproductive health and cared for their bodies in contexts characterised by multiple barriers to the health system. By focussing on the community assets of women, the article intends to contribute new perspectives on the way in which migrant health is addressed in restrictive health contexts. The study has shown that, in an environment characterised by a health system that acts to exclude, Bolivian migrant women rationally deploy a series of strategies to draw on their community assets, embodied in the networks of reciprocity of families and members of the Bolivian migrant community, as well as to the meanings of health as a natural and holistic process. The possibility of "taking advantage" of these assets leads to the development of preventive and care behaviours allowing them to more easily face the difficulties they encounter as migrants with regards to their health. In this sense, the analysis has shown, together with Menédez, that the way in which each woman experiences the health-disease-care process varies according to the knowledge and practices related to their own understandings of health, as well as the obstacles and health facilitators encountered in the search for care. The opportunity to observe the health practices of women from this perspective highlighted that the decision to use health services is often based on a conscious reflection regarding their own understanding of the body and health, as well as an evaluation of the barriers to access the health system. The article contributes to the knowledge offered by existing studies that have sought to understand the relationship of migrant women to health services, and have tended to look at women's health deficits as well as barriers to reproductive health. Despite their vulnerability, women are able to develop strategies using the resources available through their culture to mitigate the impact of barriers in the care of their body. Women choose to draw on knowledge and practices from their Andean culture, despite that they are constituted as alternatives, to avoid using health services, or to use them in combination with these knowledges and practices. Therefore, we consider that the notion of intersectionality not only contributes to understanding how women develop strategies to overcome multiple barriers, but that it should be considered for health policies designed for migration populations, to deepen understanding of different medical practices–such as some of the ones we present here–focusing on diversities (Duarte Hidalgo, 2013).

We cannot state whether migration experiences contribute to the making of flexible gender models ord the renegotiation of norms and practices concerning sexuality and reproduction. However the study critically sheds light on the way in which researchers have observed Bolivian migrant women in relation to their health, which has focused largely on how social structure impacts on health, rather than how they manage to build strategies to overcome it. We were interested in considering the way in which migrant women from Bolivia not only rely on ancestral knowledge related to healing, but in how these knowledges allow them to position themselves as agential in defence of their rights as migrants. The strengthening of reciprocal ties between members of the Bolivian community, especially amongst women, results in a dynamic exchange strengthening their capacity to face the conditions presented by the health system. This paper lies together with other studies in the field of gender and health in the region to emphasise the importance of taking the migration process as an opportunity to for women to redefine their identities in accordance with their cultural context of origin (Ariza, 2002; Pessar, 1986). To conclude, emphasis is given to the importance of incorporating a historical-political and cultural perspective in the care of migrant women that takes adequate account of their particular trajectories, the assets they possess and deploy in the host nation, and their specific needs with respect to access to health care and their cultural practices. This is a line of analysis that we will continue to deepen in future investigations.

Disclosure statement

No potential conflict of interest was reported by the authors.

Funding

This work was supported by Secretaría de Ciencia y Tecnología, Universidad Nacional de Córdoba.

References

Aizenberg, L., Rodríguez, M., & Carbonetti, A. (2015). Percepciones de los equipos de salud en torno a las mujeres migrantes bolivianas y peruanas en la ciudad de Córdoba. *Migraciones Internacionales, 8*(1), 65–94.

Álvarez, R., Moncada, M., Arias, G., Rojas, T., & Contreras, M. (2007). Rescatando el autocuidado de la salud durante el embarazo, el parto y al recién nacido: representaciones sociales de mujeres de una comunidad nativa en Perú. *Texto Contecto Enferm, 16*(4), 680–687.

Anthias, F. (2006). Belongings in a globalising and unequal world: Rethinking translocations. In N. Yuval-Davis, K. Kannabiran, & U. Vieten (Eds.), *The situated politics of belonging* (pp. 17–31). London: Sage.

Ariza, M. (2002). Migración, familia y transnacionalidad en el contexto de la globalización: Algunos puntos de reflexión. *Revista Mexicana de Sociología, 64*, 53–58.

Baeza, B. (2014). La memoria migrante y la escucha de los silencios en la experiencia del parto de mujeres migrantes bolivianas en Comodoro Rivadavia (Chubut, Argentina). *Anuario Americanista Europeo, 11*, 179–197.

Borjas, G. (1989). Economic theory and international migration. *International Migration Review, 23*, 457–485.

Caggiano, S. (2008). Que se haga cargo su país': la cultura, los Estados y el acceso a la salud de los inmigrantes bolivianos en Jujuy. In C. García Vázquez (Ed.), *Hegemonía e interculturalidad. Poblaciones originarias e inmigrantes* (pp. 243–279). Buenos Aires: Prometeo.

Cerrutti, M. (2011). *Salud y migración internacional: mujeres bolivianas en la Argentina.* Buenos Aires: PNUD- CENEP/UNFPA.

Cole, B. (2009). Gender, narratives and intersectionality: Can personal experience approaches to research contribute to "undoing gender"? *International Review of Education, 55*(5/6), 561–578.

Donato, K., Gabaccia, D., Holdaway, J., Manalasan, M., & Pessar, P. (2006). A glass half full? Gender in migration studies. *International Migration Review, 40*(1), 3–26.

Duarte Hidalgo, C. (2013). La interseccionalidad en las políticas migratorias de la Comunidad de Madrid. *Revista Punto Género, 3*, 167–194.

Goldberg, A. (2014). Trayectorias migratorias, itinerarios de salud y experiencias de participación política de mujeres migrantes bolivianas que trabajaron y vivieron en talleres textiles clandestinos del Área Metropolitana de Buenos Aires, Argentina. *Anuario Americanista Europeo, 2221-3872* (11), 199–216.

Good, B. (2003). *Medicina, Racionalidad y experiencia: una perspectiva antropológica*. Barcelona: Ediciones Belaterra.

INDEC. (2010). *Censo Nacional de Población, Hogares y Vivienda*. Buenos Aires: Instituto Nacional de Estadística y Censos.

INDEC. (2013). *Encuesta Nacional de Salud Sexual y Reproductiva*. Retrieved from http://www.indec.gob.ar/ftp/cuadros/publicaciones/enssyr_2013.pdf

Jelin, E., Grimson, A., & Zamberlin, Z. (2006). ¿Servicio?, ¿Derecho?, ¿Amenaza? La llegada de inmigrantes de países limítrofes a los servicios públicos de salud. In E. Jelin (Ed.), *Salud y migración regional. Ciudadanía, discriminación y comunicación intercultural* (pp. 27–46). Buenos Aires: Instituto de Desarrollo Económico y Social (IDES).

Lugones, M. (2008). Colonialidad y género. *Tabula Rasa, 9,* 73–101.

Magliano, M., Perissinotti, V., & Zenklusen, D. (2014). Estrategias en torno a las formas de apropiación y organización del espacio en un barrio de migrantes de la ciudad de Córdoba, Argentina. *Estudios Demográficos y Urbanos, 29,* 513–539.

Martínez Pizarro, J. (2003). *El mapa migratorio de América Latina y el Caribe. Las mujeres y el género*. Santiago de Chile: CEPAL.

Martinez Pizarro, J., & y Reboira Finardi, L. (2010). Migración, Derechos Humanos y Salud sexual y reproductiva:delicada ecuación en las fronteras. *Papeles de Población, 16*(64).

Martínez Pizarro, J., Cano, V., & Soffia, M. (2014). Tendencias y patrones de la migración latinoamericana y caribeña hacia 2010 y desafíos para una agenda regional. In *Serie Población y Desarrollo, N° 109 (LC/L.3914)* (pp. 1–72). Santiago de Chile: CEPAL.

Menéndez, E. (1985). Modelo médico hegemónico, crisis socioeconómica y estrategias de acción del sector salud. *Cuadernos Médicos Sociales, 33,* 3–34.

Menéndez, E. (2009). De racismos, esterilizaciones y algunos otros olvidos de la antropología y la epidemiología mexicanas. *Salud colectiva, 5*(2), 155–177.

Michaux, J. (2004). Hacia un sistema de salud intercultural en Bolivia: de la tolerancia a la necesidad sentida. In G. Fernández Juárez (Ed.), *Salud e interculturalidad en América Latina. Perspectivas antropológicas* (pp. 107–128). Quito: Abya-Yala.

Mora, L. (2002). *Las fronteras de la vulnerabilidad. Género, migración y derechos sexuales y reproductivos*. Santiago de Chile: UNFPA.

Organización Panamericana de la Salud. (2003). *Armonización de los Sistemas de Salud Indígenas y Sistema de Salud de las Américas. Lineamientos Estratégicos para la Incorporación de las Perspectivas, Medicinas y Terapias Indígenas en la Atención Primaria de la Salud. División de Desarrollo de Sistemas y Servicios de Salud*. Washington, DC: PAHO-WHO.

Oso, L. (1998). *Las migraciones hacia España de mujeres jefas de hogar*. Madrid: Instituto de la Mujer.

Pantelides, E., & Moreno, M. (2009). *Situación de la población en Argentina*. Buenos Aires: PNUD/UNFPA.

Pessar, P. (1986). The role of gender in Dominican settlement in the United States. In J. Nash & H. Safa (Eds.), *Women and change in Latin America* (pp. 273–294). South Hadley, MA: Bergin and Garvey.

Pessar, P., & Mahler, S. (2003). Transnational migration: Bringing gender. *International Migration Review, 37*(3), 812–846.

Rivera Cusicanqui, S. (2010). *Ch'ixinakax utxiwa: una reflexión sobre prácticas y discursos descolonizadores*. Buenos Aires: Tinta Limón.

Stolke, V. (2004). La mujer es puro cuento: la cultura del género. *Estudos Feministas, 12*(2), 77–105.

Swidler, A. (1986). Culture in action: Symbols and strategies. *American Sociological Review, 51,* 273–386.

Trigo, A. (2011). De memorias, desmemorias y antimemorias. Recuperado el 10 de marzo de 2015, de. Retrieved from http://www7.uc.cl/letras/html/6_publicaciones/pdf_revistas/taller/tl49/letras49_memorias_abril_trigo.pdf.

United Nation Fund for Population Activities (UNFPA). (2006). *Estado de la Población Mundial 2006, Hacia la Esperanza, Las Mujeres y la Migración Internacional*. New York: UNFPA.

Doctor–patient relationships amid changes in contemporary society: a view from the health communication field

Mónica Petracci, Patricia K. N. Schwarz, Victoria I. Ma. Sánchez Antelo and
Ana María Mendes Diz

ABSTRACT

Synopsis: In this article, we propose to understand the doctor–patient relationship (DPR) using a health communications perspective, as it is located in the sociohistorical framework of modernising processes. The paper analyses the academic literature about the doctor-patient relationship (DPR) during the period of 1980–2015, gathered from key words in digital collections and indexed magazines available in three electronic databases (SISBI, SciELO and DIALNET). Eighty-four articles were selected from the initial search. The results suggest three axes of thematisation of the DPR over the period analysed: patient satisfaction, models of relationship between professionals and patients, and eHealth. The latter, eHealth, demonstrates the current transformation of social and communication order and is the main axis of reflection and investigation.

Introduction

In health consultations, periodic health checks, searches for health information, treatments, diagnostics, and prevention, among others, health professionals and patients build a relationship that oscillates between two typical models: one close to paternalism and focused on the doctor's authority; and another that recognises the patient's autonomy. Although it is true that such models differ, the doctor-patient relationship (DPR) is an asymmetrical social relationship whose main points of support are the difference of knowledge (Boltansky, 1975), of language and vocabulary (Clavreul, 1978) and of power (Foucault, 1953/2001).

Interest in the link between doctors and patients, or between doctors and the sick, has a long history (Laín Entralgo, 1964) and has received extensive academic attention from a range of disciplines (History of Medicine, Medical Sciences, Social Sciences, Anthropology). The questions that guide the exploration and description of this academic attention focuses on communication: Is communication understood as a tool for the purposes of navigating a face-to-face individual relationship? Does it seek to understand the asymmetries of that social relationship?

Our theoretical approach to the DPR from the field of health communications understands that communication is not a mere transmission of information from a professional to a patient. It is a complex process in which other actors participate (Cuberli & Araujo, 2015; Del Pozo, Román, Alcántara, & Domínguez, 2015; Obregón & Waisbord, 2012; Petracci, 2015; Petracci & Waisbord, 2011; Rogers, 1996) in the context of contemporary social and communication changes (Bauman, 2003, 2007; Beck, 1998; Rosa, 2011).

This article has four sections: communication and health: a focus on DPR; methodology; axes of thematisation of the DPR; conclusions and discussion. The paper analyses the academic literature about the doctor-patient relationship (DPR) during the period of 1980–2015, gathered from key words in digital collections and indexed magazines available in three electronic databases (SISBI, SciELO and DIALNET).

Health communication: a focus on DPR

Health communication is (in a Bourdeausian sense) an interdisciplinary field, academically established in the United States and some European countries in the second half of the twentieth century. It is heterogeneous due to the diverse range of issues present at its intersection (Petracci & Waisbord, 2011): the disease in the individual and collective identity construction; health as an agenda and the construction of hegemony; the risk of epidemics and the need to communicate messages of prevention, the demands of rights, care and research in health as an axis of social mobility; and health–disease as news in the media, the social networks and consultation fora.

The DPR is also placed at that juncture. It is understood as a type of interaction materially and symbolically anchored that includes, on the one hand, links of dispute and relational power and, on the other, a departure from the position that reduces communication to the learning of skills on how professionals must conduct themselves with the patients, or it is guided by an 'instrumental utility' (Del Pozo et al., 2015, p. 11).

Following Rosa (2011), contemporary processes of rationalisation, differentiation, society-nature, individuation and acceleration, helps to understand the complexities of changes in the DPR from the communications field. These include the prioritising of the bureaucratic rationality of health systems over face-to-face ties and relationships; the patient's transformation into a consuming client who, in addition, can become a producer of health knowledges; the anonymity and emphasis on the provisional ties with professionals; the presence of risks in consultations linked to prevention; the crisis of the normative structures in which the relationship between health professionals and patients evolve linked with eclectic forms of care; and the increase in workload on professionals, which can generate perceptions of dissatisfaction about the duration of the consultation for patients and professionals.

Methodology

We used two methodological stages to retrieve literature for this analysis:

(1) The search for digital collections and indexed magazines available in electronic data-bases, and national and international sources. Three key words were used: doctor-patient relationship (DPR), eHealth, and gender. The research was conducted by the Gino Germani Research Institute's Documentation Centre.[1] The following libraries were consulted, based on the search strategies and the use of registries for each source focusing on the key words: the Faculties of Social Sciences, Medicine, and the Gino Germani Research Institute's Documentation Centre (Buenos Aires University) in SISBI (Information and Libraries System of the Buenos Aires University)[2]; as well as the SciELO (Scientific Electronic Library Online); and DIALNET databases (each database is defined in Table 1). From the initial search, which was not tabulated by the type of database, we selected 98 results through consensus with the research team.

(2) Definition of inclusion criteria in the final sample required that the article pre-sented the findings of an empirical investigation, or developed theoretical reflec-tions, or gave practical recommendations. Fourteen publications were excluded from the initial selection during this stage. The final sample consisted of 84 publications.

Axes of thematisation of the DPR

Exploration of the retrieved articles were guided by two hypotheses. The first refers to the impact of technological changes to the DPR: eHealth displays different modalities and produces positive and negative changes in the traditional face-to-face relationship between doctors and patients (modalities such as online searches before or after the con-sultation, participation in online fora, sending tests results via email, and telemedicine, among others). The second hypothesis refers to the characteristics of the change process: the changes produced by eHealth coexist with previous formats, and do not sub-stitute them. In this context, the Internet is an *a la carte* communicative medium set according to the tastes and needs of each user, ending the separation between audio-visual and printed media, popular and erudite culture and, entertainment and information (Castells, 1999; Mattelart, 1996).

The following paragraphs discuss the selected axes: patient satisfaction, models of doctor–patient relationship and eHealth.

Table 1. Description of literature databases.

Literature databases	
SISBI	A system that coordinates, promotes, and leads the cooperation between Units of Information of the Libraries' System of the University of Buenos Aires to provide excellent services and products to different users, and encourage continuous capacitation.
SciELO	Online scientific library for the cooperative electronic publications of scientific magazines in the Internet, especially developed to answer the needs of scientific communication in the developing countries, especially from Latin America and the Caribbean.
DIALNET	Library cooperation project initiated at the La Rioja University, Spain, which collects and provides access mostly to documents published in Spain in any language, published in Spanish in any country or that deal with Hispanic topics.

Source: Created by the authors.

Patient satisfaction

Patient satisfaction was selected as a theme due to its presence in the retrieved articles of our sample during the 1980s and 1990s, and for the weight assigned to the communicational dimension (understood as learning abilities) for the patient to express a greater level of satisfaction regarding the relationship with the doctor and the health system.

A trend here focussed on the factors that produce satisfaction (such as empathy, treatment and trust, continuity (or not) with a same professional) and those that would hinder it (barriers to cultural accessibility, loss of the personal dimension in the clinical model for new diagnostic and therapeutic resources) (Bianconi, 1988; Climent y Mendes Diz, 1986; Donoso-Sabando, 2014; Florenzano, 1986; Martínez Salgado y Leal, 2003; Orellana-Peña, 2008; Prece, Necchi, Adamo, & Schufer, 1988; Rodríguez, 2006; Schufer, 1983). Other topics outlined included the interaction of social determinants (Duarte Nunes, 1989; Ong, de Haes, Hoos, & Lammes, 1995) and the impact of communication on patient's satisfaction and adherence to treatments (Cófreces, Ofman, & Stefani, 2014; Moore et al., 2004).

Regarding the differences in satisfaction in relation to the gender of health professionals, Ainsworth-Vaughin (1998) uses a sociolinguistics approach. Hall, Irish, Roter, Ehrlich, and Miller (1994) analyse the relationship between doctors and patients (men and women) in terms of verbal and non-verbal communication in one-hundred medical consultations. They found different patterns, especially in non-verbal communication. The relationship between female doctors and women patients is the one that offers greater contrast than with the relationship between women doctors and male patients. The authors found that, compared to their male counterparts, women doctors often had friendlier attitudes and behaviour that built a participative scenario for the patients, which was associated with greater levels of satisfaction. Cooper-Patrick et al. (1999) argue that the studies focused on investigating the influence of gender of the patients in the medical consultation showed that the aspects that give more satisfaction (answer to the request for information and allocated time) are accentuated in female patients and professionals. Roter, Hall, and Aoki (2002) found that that more than their male counterparts, female primary care doctors displayed a communication centred on the patient.

Other retrieved articles, which linked satisfaction with the quality of attention received by patients (Donabedian, 1991), were focussed on conceptualising and measuring the levels of satisfaction. These challenged the validity of other studies given the problems that the concept of pre-existing 'expectations' presents to measurement of satisfaction, theoretically and methodologically, given that satisfaction is related to expectations (Necchi, 1998). Regarding the modernising processes of Rosa (2011), rationalisation and acceleration are also related with this axis of patient satisfaction. Although the first studies incorporated technology and standardisation of care and diagnosis processes, they also excluded components that can limit a patient's satisfaction, such as affective and direct treatment. Regarding acceleration in the organisational components that favour or disadvantage satisfaction, one can recognise a multiplicity of temporalities for patients (allocation of appointments, delivery of studies, etc.), as well as the commodification of health systems on the actors that comprise it (Donabedian, 1991; Ong et al., 1995).

Relationship models

Historically, the description and analysis of relationship models has attracted interest among studies in this field. Also, because it expresses the passage from a paternalistic model into a more autonomist one in the 'stage' of the DPR (Bohórquez, 2004).

For Lázaro and Gracia (2006, p. 7) it meant a transformation 'with scarce historical precedents'. Traditionally a passive receptor of the doctor's decisions, the patient as understood at the end of the twentieth century transformed into an agent with rights and the capacity for autonomous decision over therapeutic and diagnostic procedures. The doctor's position moved from a paternal figure to become more of a technical advisor of his/her patients, who are offered knowledge and advice but who are no longer obliged to take the doctor's decision. The emergence of other actors and greater horizontal ties joined the bipolar and vertical clinical relationship. These changes are complex and conflictive processes that were developed within a framework of the transformations and challenges of the medical profession (Llovet, 1999; Oriol Bosch & Pardell Alenta, 2004).

Like the previous axis, the retrieved articles here refered to the acquisition of abilities and formulation of communicational recommendations in the different models (Clèries Costa et al., 2003; Cordella, 2004; Fahy & Smith, 1999; García et al., 1995; Gordon & Sterling Edwards, 1995; Korsch & Harding, 1998; Ruiz Moral, Rodríguez, & Epstein, 2003; Vidal y Benito, 2002) and, unlike the previous axis of patient satisfaction, this literature represents a critical communicational approach (Barry, Stevenson, Britten, Barber, & Bradley, 2001; Epstein, 2006; Gumucio-Dagron, 2010; Ong et al., 1995; Rodríguez Arce, 2008; Roter & Hall, 2006).

The literature on relationships also includes the assessment of patient autonomy in medical decision-making (De Benedetti Zunino, Pastor Carvajal, & Bandrés Sánchez, 2006); the participation of patients (Thompson, 2007); and reflects on the DPR and the problems of communication of the 'truth', and human rights (Gajardo Ugás, 2009; Ocampo-Martínez, 2002; Sánchez González, 2007; Skirbekk, Middelthon, Hjortdahl, & Finset, 2011) from other perspectives such as bioethics and psychology (Mucci, 2007).

Regarding the modernising processes of Rosa (2011), the individuation and differentiation are related to this axis. With regards to individualisation–a result of social fragmentation and atomization–the focus of the studies included in this axis emphasise the individual performance of doctors. On the other hand, structural and functional differentiation refers to the lack of social cohesion and, hence, the privatisation of risks, and the socialisation in provisional links including the one established between the patient with the doctor.

Ehealth: internet as support and a social actor

We chose this set of literature due to its centrality of the New Information and Communication Technologies (NICTs) for national health systems, and for the relationships between the health system's actors (such as the DPR). eHealth has been the subject of one systematic review (Pagliari et al., 2005) and it has been an ongoing presence in the literature since the year 2000.

In this literature eHealth (or health online or *telesalud*) seems to comprise consultation practices and publication of information, diffusion, interaction, and online health care. An agreed definition, however, is subject of debate. Some authors link the DRP to the use of the New Information and Communications Technologies (NICTs) in general, and the internet in particular. The access by patients to information regarding online health is a topic of much attention early on (Barnes et al., 2003; Broom, 2005; Kivits, 2006; Lupiá-ñez-Villanueva, 2008; Marín-Torres et al., 2013; Nwosu & Cox, 2000; Rahmqvist & Bara, 2007; Wathen & Harris, 2007).

Andreassen, Trondsen, Kummervold, Gammon, and Hjortdahl (2006) observe that trust in online interactions between doctors and patients is built according to postmodern standards, as it is in other social relationships, and that patient's need for trust in the professionals and the health system are key to understand the use of the NTICs by patients. Jacobson (2007) uses a Medline review to analyse how the internet impact on the consultation (as a reason for discussion that challenges medical authority) and the empowering experience of patients. Using a trend analysis of three population studies carried out in Sweden in 2002, 2003 and 2005, Rahmqvist and Bara (2007) show that there was a significant increase in internet use during the period studied and that the predictors for its use as a source of information were age, sex, perceived health, area of residence and the type of medical encounter (first or repeated).

Wathen and Harris (2007) interviewed women living in rural areas of Canada regarding their experiences on the search of information and health given the major difficulties of access to health by people living far away from large urban centres. The government sought to empower patients and encourage processes of selfcare in health through online information as a way to overcome distance difficulties, and the findings demonstrate that seeking information online provides emotional sharing by allowing dialogue between people with similar experiences. Later, we observe that some authors of eHealth literature reflect about the DPR and internet in structural terms and fully addressing the functioning logics of the health system. Jung and Berthon (2009) developed a theoretical reflection regarding health care through the internet; and argue that it is a useful resource amid the growing demand for care due to the progressive ageing of the population.

Laakso, Armstrong, and Usher (2012) consider how a virtual platform that addresses health demands online should be constituted. In that same line of inquiry, Lustria, Smith, and Hinnant (2011) questioned the relationship between social inequalities and access to health services online. Armstrong, Koteyko, and Powell (2012) analysed an online forum of diabetic patients in England, which the authors propose can be an alternative for health systems that face ageing populations and the costs associated with the care of long term illnesses. This concern around the access to health information online remains current (Chiu, 2011; Stern, Cotten, & Drentea, 2012).

With the advance of technology we find retrieved articles that refer to the greater complexity in the use of the internet such as the analysis of online heath care practices (Bert, Passi, Scaioli, Gualano, & Siliquini, 2016; Kim, 2015; Rodríguez, Almeida, & Valdés, 2013; Wilkowska & Ziefle, 2012). Bert et al. (2016) analysed online applications for tablets and smartphones for pregnancies and childbirth, and found that most of the applications do not explicitly state the origin of the information or guarantee the preservation of privacy of the information required for the subscription. This concern for the handling of health information online is continuing (Kim, 2015).

In relation to Rosa's (2001) references to modernising processes and rationalizations, which are now currently characterised by flexible processes of control, this has gone hand in hand with New Information and Communication Technologies (NICTs). The third modernising process is also present and refers to the relationship of the social to nature. The author interprets the work of transforming the nature of subjects as a production of means of life and, at the same time, of themselves.

Conclusions and discussion

This section is organised to consider (1) the theoretical approach taken in the existing research; (2) the methodological design; (3) the findings from the analyses; and (4) some final cosiderations.

1. In this article, we reflect upon the DPR from the field of Health Communication. Health communication contributed to differentiate communication as a tool intended to recommend how the DPR link should be and as a theoretical approach through which to build the concept and establish practice. It is not about transforming the communicational recommendations in theoretical discoveries that forget the reality in which the DPR takes place, nor formulating a binary approach that ends up overshadowing what is sought to clarify. Instead, it formulates recommendations that, on the one hand, involve the patient-citizen with health as a right, autonomy, patient's participation in the decisions concerning his/her body and in the communication of diagnostics and treatments, interculturality, media and virtual platforms understood as social resources (Waisbord, 2015, p. 143); and, on the other hand, the challenges that modernising processes pose to the health system and its actors.

2. The initial search presented idiomatic limitations; technical (systematization difficulties), and search words. For search words, 'eHealth' and 'DPR' were the most appropriate. Nevertheless, in the case of 'eHealth', our evaluation shows that it would have been also convenient to accompany the concept with other specific types of use (consultation fora, information search, mobile-phone applications, among others).

The sample in this study is not representative. We do not seek to make generalisations of all the findings from this type of study. Despite those limitations, and in addition to the ones already pointed out regarding the search, we consider that the contribution of the readings and the analysis of the articles was to explore the initial questions from the field of communicational health.

3. Taking into account the reflective view of this article, the limitations of the search and the scope of the aforementioned literature, we believe that that our analysis reveals the transformation of the paternalistic model of DPR into another leaning towards patient autonomy. eHealth has played an important role of this process of change around DPR: positive change because it favours access to information and the autonomy of the patient, and negative change because the information can be of poor quality or outdated; because it opens a spectrum of exposure and control of personal information turned into virtual sites, as well as a technological update that involves patients, professionals and other actors of the health system.

The axes–patient's satisfaction, models of relationship between professionals and patients, and eHealth–are interrelated and do not exclude new axes derived from analyses guided by other theoretical frameworks and research experiences.

The patient's satisfaction is related to the perception of availability and empathy of the health professional, independently from the DPR model to which the physician ascribes, and of the practice and the personal or online media through which they communicate. On the other hand, the professional's satisfaction is related to changes in the DPR which, as the initial asymmetry dissipates, confront doctors with excess of information by patients, often from unreliable sources.

The DPR model seem to have gone through transformations: from paternalistic and hierarchical to one with more patient autonomy; from one that positions patients as passive ill people to a subject with agency, capacity and with rights; from a dyadic format to an institutional one in which the patient is a user of plural services in more than one institution; from a direct link to another mediated by technology and the internet; from a relationship where the doctor's word was unquestionable to another where the patient is allowed to doubt health professionals, negotiate the diagnosis and treatment, or is allowed to discuss and/or complain to government authorities, consumer associations, and lodge complaints, or lawsuits.

These changes do not replace but coexist with previous formats (although not without conflict) depending on each health situation and on the required levels of complexity. These changes also depend on the characteristics of the care system, and the degree of empowerment of the patient, among other things. The communicational dimension, in these changes, was valued regarding the secondary place assigned by the biomedical model. The articles of focus in this paper go through different, yet non-exclusive, paths where the communicational dimension is posed as an individual technical skill favouring the DPR and adherence to treatment, or is presented as an area from which social issues such as power, culture and socioeconomic differences become evident.

The 1980s literature included in our analyses describe patient passivity as a condition that is taken for granted and not questioned or analysed. It is seen to be part of the basic conditions in which biomedicine should operate in a 'normal' scenario. We noted that the focus in the literature with patient satisfaction was a seed upon which, combined with other phenomena such as advances in terms of rights, greater access to information, need for the profitability of the health service, development of the communication technology, among others, was reconfigured into greater spaces of action for patients. Patient satisfaction became relevant to medical training, among other issues, which had traditionally been monopolised by biomedical knowledge exclusively. These processes intervene in the modes of care and treatment, as well as of communication between doctors and patients. Table 2 presents a synthesis of the transformations in DPR registered in the literature reviewed in this article.

The axis eHealth has a strong presence with the spread of globalisation and the development of NICTs (Osorio, 2011). It is inseparable from the patient satisfaction since the changes in the DPR model are scenarios in which it excels. The articles in this paper show the interest that the search for online health information produces as a subject of study, the explicit or implicit presence as well as the influence of that information sought online by the patients in the traditional sense of the DPR. That this search contributes to a fluid interaction will depend on the interests and knowledge of the health system's actors. The most recent articles address the logic of operating online virtual health care platforms. They propose to develop both instances of computer and internet use learning for patients

Table 2. Synthesis of the process of transformation in the doctor-patient relationship.

Paternalistic Model	Transformations of the paternalistic model towards an autonomous model
A receiving patient is passive to medical decisions.	Based on an agent patient with defined rights and decision autonomy over the diagnostic and therapeutic procedures.
Concern for the patient's satisfaction is based on the legitimacy of the doctor's power and its hegemonic expert knowledge.	Concern for patient's satisfaction based on the legitimacy of medical power due to expert knowledge *and* the consideration of technological, communicational, and bioethical changes.
Doctor training fully biomedical	Doctor training happens with participation of patients.
Professional training based on expert knowledge to be exercised through a vertical, paternalistic, and authoritarian model.	Professional training based on the expert knowledge to be exercised from a more horizontal model, with diversity of specialised knowledge and bioethical principles.
DPRs within the framework of systems with emphasis on rational bureaucratic criteria.	DPRs in the framework of systems with an emphasis on economist criteria.
Doctor-patient relationships in the framework of consultations with longer duration.	DPRs in the framework of consultations of shorter duration based in the contemporary process of acceleration.
Greater autonomy of the doctor.	Less autonomy of doctor as result of a greater control over medical practice by the State, patient organisations, supranational institutions, and the market, among others.
Less power for the patient	Greater power for the patient as result of access to information, rights, democratic practices, mechanisms of collective organisation of patients, development of ethical and legal control of the medical practices, among others. This process generates the possibility of change and resistance to the control devises over the body of users of the health system.
	Internet. Google. eHealth
Difficult access to medical information	Easier access to medical information
Scarce search for medical information	Search for medical information in websites and consultation fora.
Very little discussion with the doctor.	Increase in the discussions and decisions negotiated with the doctor.

Source: created by the authors.

and physicians, such as learning about procedures and devices, so that the access to information and health care is efficient and reaches as many users as possible. Yet, no article we reviewed questions the current and future existence of this actor/support –eHealth–, which shows the current sociocommunicational transformations and is, currently, the main axis of reflection and research.

One limitation regarding eHealth in this search is concern about patient involvement. A recent review by Barello et al. (2016) addresses the role of eHealth in people's participation in health care by considering matters of subjectivity s (ie emotional, cognitive and behavioural), and conclude that the interventions aimed at each component individually, instead of considering the complexity of the psychological processes.

The focus on the DPR by the field of health communication in modernising processes in this review revealed that communication is understood as a tool at the service of an individual face-to-face relationship fundamentally in the patient satisfaction axis. In contrast, this view coexists with a more critical one that seeks to understand the relationship's asymmetries in the models' axis. In the last axis, eHealth, communication is placed in the technological context of contemporary society and renews the debate about patient's autonomy in the face of eHealth experiences because, although eHealth broadens possibilities for health care, it also renews mechanisms of social control and contributes to the persistence of access difficulties.

Table 3. Facilitators and obstacles of the doctor-patient relationship.

Facilitators	Obstacles
Empathy/Affectivity	Specific technical language
Information on the internet	Information on the internet
Empowerment of the patient	Power of the doctor
Organisation of patients' networks	Economic rationalism in health care
Rights of the patients	Abuse of legal litigation towards medical practice
Medical attention through the internet	Lack of legislation protecting the diffusion of patients' medical information.
Training of doctors with participation of patients.	Lack of time in the consultation
Preoccupation with patient satisfaction.	Technological mediation and impersonality

Source: created by the authors.

From the analysis of the emerging axes aspects develop which we classify due to their facilitating or obstructing character of the DPR (see Table 3). The outlined classification is not rigid and acknowledges the complexity of defining an aspect as an obstacle and/or facilitator. For instance, the collective organisation of patients help in the quality of health care. However, sometimes it conflicts with the DPR because it questions medical knowledge and practice (Armstrong et al., 2012). Accessing health information online favours the patient and permits a deeper and more fluent communication with doctors. Yet, this depends on the type of medical specialty. The facilitating character of the internet is also relative because inequity in access to technology deepens social gaps (Lustria et al., 2011). Yet, on the other hand, patients' internet use can overload the health system due to the confusion it generates (Nwosu & Cox, 2000). Social and economic gaps are influential here. According to González (2008), the relation between the size of a country's Gross Domestic Product (GDP) and the density of installed technology are directly proportional. NICTs assume equal standing in access and capacity of individual to use technology. Those without access and capacity experience further marginalisation (Castells, 1999).

4. We conclude that the communicational dimension of health–understood as a complex process–within the framework of modernising processes is a view that contributes to understanding the changes produced in the DPR, which favour or obstruct the fluidity of the relationship. eHealth establishes a trade-off for the DPR: although it distances patients from the paternalistic tutelage of doctors, it generates needs among patients for training to better exercise those practices. Furthermore, it also challenges the decision of professionals and patients, and of health systems facing health care in a context of technological changes.

Notes

1. *Centro de Documentación del Instituto de Investigaciones Gino Germani.*
2. *Sistema de Bibliotecas y de Información de la Universidad de Buenos Aires.*

Disclosure statement

No potential conflict of interest was reported by the authors.

References

Ainsworth-Vaughin, N. (1998). *Claiming power in doctor patient talk*. New York: Oxford University Press.

Andreassen, H. K., Trondsen, M., Kummervold, P. E., Gammon, D., & Hjortdahl, P. (2006). Patients who use e-mediated communication with their doctor: New constructions of trust in the patient-doctor relationship. *Qualitative Health Research, 16*(2), 238–248.

Armstrong, N., Koteyko, N., & Powell, J. (2012). «Oh dear, should I really be saying that on here?»: Issues of identity and authority in an online diabetes community. *Health: An Interdisciplinary Journal for the Social Study of Health, Illness and Medicine, 16*(4), 347–365.

Barello, S., Triberti, S., Graffigna, G., Libreri, C., Serino, S., Hibbard, J., & Riva, G. (2016). eHealth for patient engagement: A systematic review. *Frontiers in Psychology, 6,* 850. doi:10.3389/fpsyg. 2015.02013

Barnes, M., Penrod, C., Neiger, B., Merrill, R., Thackeray, R., Eggett, D., & Thomas, E. (2003). Measuring the relevance of evaluation criteria among health information seekers on the internet. *Journal of Health Psychology, 8*(1), 71–82.

Barry, C. A., Stevenson, F. A., Britten, N., Barber, N., & Bradley, C. P. (2001). Giving voice to the lifeworld. More humane, more effective medical care? A qualitative study of doctor–patient communication in general practice. *Social Science and Medicine, 53,* 487–505.

Bauman, Z. (2003). *Modernidad Líquida*. Buenos Aires: Fondo de Cultura Económica.

Bauman, Z. (2007). *Tiempos líquidos. Vivir en una época de incertidumbre*. Barcelona: Tusquets.

Beck, U. (1998). *La sociedad del riesgo: hacia una nueva modernidad*. Barcelona: Paidós.

Bert, F., Passi, S., Scaioli, G., Gualano, M., & Siliquini, R. (2016). There comes a baby! What should I do? Smartphones' pregnancy-related applications: A web-based overview. *Health Informatics Journal, 22*(3), 608–617.

Bianconi, Z. (1988). Porqué se quejan los pacientes. *Medicina y sociedad, 11*(1/2), 25–29.

Bohórquez, F. (2004). El diálogo como mediador de la relación medico - paciente. *Revista Electrónica de la Red de Investigación Educativa, 1*(1), (Julio-Diciembre). Disponible en http://revista.iered.org

Boltansky, L. (1975). *Los usos sociales del cuerpo*. Buenos Aires: Periferia.

Broom, A. (2005). Medical specialists' accounts of the impact of the internet on the doctor-patient relationship. *Health: An Interdisciplinary Journal for the Social Study of Health, Illness and Medicine, 9*(3), 319–338.

Castells, M. (1999). *La era de la información. Economía, sociedad y cultura. Volumen I. La sociedad red*. Buenos Aires: Siglo XXI.

Chiu, Y.-C. (2011). Probing, impelling, but not offending doctors: The role of the internet as an information source for patients' interactions with doctors. *Qualitative Health Research, 21*(12), 1658–1666.

Clavreul, J. (1978). No existe relación médico paciente. *Cuadernos Médico Sociales. Asociación Médica de Rosario*, Argentina, 7(marzo), 32–50.

Clèries Costa, X., Borrell Carrió, F., Epstein, R. M., Kronfly Rubianoa, E., Escoda Arestéa, J. J., & Martínez-Carretero, J. M. (2003). Aspectos comunicacionales: el reto de la competencia de la profesión médica. *Atención Primaria, 32*(2), 110–117.

Climent, G. y Mendes Diz, A. M. (1986). Accesibilidad cultural: Satisfacción de las necesidades en la relación-médico-paciente. *Revista Internacional de Medicina Familiar, 3*(4), 8–13.

Cooper-Patrick, L., Gallo, J., Gonzales, J., Vu, H., Powe, N., & Nelson, C. (1999). Race, gender and partnership in the patient-physician relationship. *JAMA, 282*(6), 583–589.

Cordella, M. (2004). *The dynamic consultation: A discourse analytical study of doctor–patient communication*. Pragmatics and Beyond New Series, Volume 28. Amsterdam: John Benjamins Publishing Company.

Cófreces, P., Ofman, S., & Stefani, D. (2014). La comunicación en la relación médico-paciente. Análisis de la literatura científica entre 1990 y 2010. *Revista de Comunicación y Salud, 4,* 19–34.

Cuberli, M., & Araujo, I. (2015). Las prácticas de la comunicación y salud: intersecciones e intersticios. In *La salud en la trama comunicacional contemporánea* (pp. 21–33). Buenos Aires: Prometeo. M. Petracci (Coord.), 2015.

De Benedetti Zunino, M. E., Pastor Carvajal, S. M., & Bandrés Sánchez, M. P. (2006). Evaluación de la autonomía del paciente en el proceso de la toma de decisiones médicas. *Revista Medica Herediana*, *17*(1), 21–27.

Del Pozo, J., Román, A., Alcántara, R. y Domínguez, M. (2015). *Medios de comunicación y salud.* Sevilla: Astigi.

Donabedian, A. (1991). Una aproximación a la monitorización de la calidad asistencial. *Control de Calidad Asistencial*, *6*(2), 1–6, 31–39.

Donoso-Sabando, C. (2014). La empatía en la relación médico-paciente como manifestación del respeto por la dignidad de la persona. *Persona y Bioética*, *18*(2), 184–193.

Duarte Nunes, E. (1989). Relación Médico Paciente y sus determinanates sociales. *Cuadernos médico sociales*, *48*, 29–38.

Epstein, R. M. (2006). Making communication research matter: What do patients notice, what do patients want, and what do patients need? *Patient Education and Counseling*, *60*(3), 272–278.

Fahy, K., & Smith, P. (1999). From the sick role to subject position: A new approach to the medical encounter. *Health: An Interdisciplinary Journal for the Social Study of Health, Illness and Medicine*, *3*(1), 71–94.

Florenzano, R. (1986). La relación médico paciente en la medicina familiar. *Revista Internacional de Medicina Familiar*, *3*(4), 23–27.

Foucault, M. (1953/2001). *El nacimiento de la clínica. Una arqueologia de la mirada médica.* Buenos Aires: Siglo XXI.

Gajardo Ugás, A. (2009). La comunicación de la verdad en la relación médico-paciente terminal. *Acta bioethica*, *15*(2), 212–215.

García, D., Rucker, S., de Kerschen, S., Arguello, M., Ustarroz, F., & Pérez, G. (1995). La comunicación en la relación médico paciente. *Claves en Medicina y Psicoanálisis*, Abril, Número, *7*, 20–22.

González, J. (2008). Digitalizados por decreto: ciberculturas o inclusión forzada en América Latina. *En: Estudios sobre las culturas contemporáneas*, *XIV*(27), 47–76. México: Universidad de Colima.

Gordon, T., & Sterling Edwards, W. (1995). *Making the patient your partner: Communication skills for doctors and others caregivers.* Westport: GreenWood Publishing Group.

Gumucio-Dagron, A. (2010). Cuando el doctor no sabe. Comentarios críticos sobre promoción de la salud. Comunicación y Participación. *Época II. Estudios sobre las Culturas Contemporáneas*, *XVI*(31), 67–93.

Hall, J., Irish, J., Roter, D., Ehrlich, C., & Miller, L. (1994). Gender in medical encounters: An analysis of physician and patient communication in a primary care setting. *Health Psychology*, *13*(5), 384–392.

Jacobson, P. (2007). Empowering the physician-patient relationship: The effect of the internet. *Partnership: The Canadian Journal of Library and Informatiion Practice and Research*, *2*(1), 1–13.

Jung, M.-L., & Berthon, P. (2009). Fulfilling the promise: A model for delivering successful online health care. *Journal of Medical Marketing*, *9*(3), 243–254.

Kim, Y.-M. (2015). Is seeking health information online different from seeking general information online? *Journal of Information Science*, *41*(2), 228–241.

Kivits, J. (2006). Informed patients and the internet: A mediated context for consultations with health professionals. *Journal of Health Psychology*, *11*(2), 269–282.

Korsch, B., & Harding, C. (1998). *The intelligent patient's guide to doctor patient relationship.* New York: Oxford University Press.

Laakso, E.-L., Armstrong, K., & Usher, W. (2012). Cyber-management of people with chronic disease: A potential solution to eHealth challenges. *Health Education Journal*, *71*(4), 483–490.

Laín Entralgo, P. (1964). *La relación médico enfermo. Historia y teoría.* Madrid: Revista de Occidente.

Lázaro, J. y Gracia, D. (2006). La relación médico-enfermo a través de la historia. *Anales del Sistema Sanitario de Navarra*, *29*(3), 7–17.

Llovet, J. (1999). Transformaciones en la profesión médica. un cuadro de situación al final del siglo. En *Salud, cambio social y política. Perspectivas desde América Latina* (pp. 335–349). México DF: EDAMEX.

Lupiáñez-Villanueva, F. (2008). *Internet, Salud y Sociedad. Análisis de los usos de Internet relacionados con la Salud en Catalunya*. Barcelona: UOC.

Lustria, M. L. A., Smith, S. A., & Hinnant, C. (2011). Exploring digital divides: An examination of eHealth technology use in health information seeking, communication and personal health information management in the USA. *Health Informatics Journal*, *17*(3), 224–243.

Marín-Torres, V., Valverde Aliaga, J., Sánchez Miró, I., Sáenz del Castillo Vicente, M. I., Polentinos-Castro, E. y Garrido, B. A. (2013). Internet como fuente de información sobre salud en pacientes de atención primaria y su influencia en la relación médico-paciente. *Atención Primaria*, *45*(1), 46–53.

Martínez Salgado, C. y Leal, G. (2003). Sobre la calidad clínica de la atención: El problema de la relación médico-paciente. *Anales Médicos*, *48*(4), 242–254.

Mattelart, A. (1996) *La Comunicación-Mundo. Historia de las ideas y de las estrategias*. México DF: Siglo XXI.

Moore, P., Sickel, A., Malat, J., Williams, D., Jackson, J., & Adler, N. (2004). Psychosocial factors in medical and psychological treatment avoidance: The role of the doctor-patient relationship. *Journal of Health Psychology*, *9*(3), 421–433.

Mucci, M. (2007). La Relación Medico-Paciente ¿un Vínculo Distinto O Distante? *Psicodebate. Psicología, Cultura y Sociedad*, *8*, 61–78.

Necchi, S. (1998). Los usuarios como protagonistas. *Medicina y Sociedad e Insituto Universitario CEMIC*, 1–15.

Nwosu, C. R., & Cox, B. (2000). The impact of the Internet on the doctor-patient relationship. *Health Informatics Journal*, *6*, 156–161.

Obregón, R., & Waisbord, S. (2012). *The handbook of global health communication*. Hoboken, NJ: Wiley- Blackwell.

Ocampo-Martínez, J. (2002). La bioética y la relación Médico-Paciente. *Cirugía y Cirujanos*, *70*(1), 55–59.

Ong, L., de Haes, J., Hoos, A., & Lammes, F. (1995). Doctor-patient communication: A review of the literature. *Social Science and Medicine*, *40*(7), 903–918.

Orellana-Peña, C. (2008). Intimidad del paciente, pudor y educación médica. *Persona y Bioética*, *12*(1), 8–15.

Oriol Bosch, A. y Pardell Alenta, H. (2004). *El nuevo profesionalismo médico: una ideología expresada en conductas*. Monografías Humanitas 7. Barcelona: Fundación Medicina y Humanidades Médicas.

Osorio, J. (2011). Evolution and changes in the physician-patient relationship. *Colombia Médica*, *42*(3), 400–405.

Pagliari, C., Sloan, D., Gregor, P., Sullivan, F., Detmer, D., Kahan, J. P., … MacGillivray, S. (2005). What is eHealth (4): A scoping exercise to map the field. *Journal of Medical Internet Research*, *7*, e9. doi:10.2196/jmir.7.1.e9

Petracci, M. (2015). *La salud en la trama comunicacional contemporánea* (1.ª ed.). Buenos Aires: Prometeo.

Petracci, M. y Waisbord, S. (2011). *Comunicación y salud en la Argentina* (1.ª ed.). Buenos Aires: La Crujía.

Prece, G., Necchi, S., Adamo, M. y Schufer, M. (1988). Estrategias familiares frente a la atención de la salud. *Medicina y sociedad*, *11*(1/2), 2–11.

Rahmqvist, M., & Bara, A.-C. (2007). Patients retrieving additional information via the internet: A trend analysis in a Swedish population, 2000–05. *Scandinavian Journal of Public Health*, *35*(5), 533–539.

Rodríguez, S., Almeida, J. y Valdés, F. (2013). Relación médico paciente y la eSalud. *Revista Cubana de Investigaciones Biomédicas*, *32*(4), 411–420.

Rodríguez, H. (2006). La relación médico-paciente. *Revista Cubana de Salud Pública, 32*(4), 2–13.

Rodríguez Arce, M. (2008). *Relación Médico-Paciente*. La Habana: Editorial Ciencias Médicas.

Rogers, E. M. (1996). The field of health communication today: An up-to-date report. *Journal of Health Communication, 1*, 15–24.

Rosa, H. (2011). Aceleración social: consecuencias éticas y políticas de una sociedad de alta velocidad desincronizada. *Persona y Sociedad, XXV*(1), 9–49.

Roter, D., Hall, J., & Aoki, Y. (2002). Physician gender effects in medical communication. *JAMA, 288*(6), 756–764.

Roter, D., & Hall, J. (2006). *Doctors talking with patients/ patients talking with doctors: Improving communication in medical visits* (2nd ed.). Westport: Praeger.

Ruiz Moral, R., Rodríguez, J. y Epstein, R. (2003). ¿Qué estilo de consulta debería emplear con mis pacientes? Reflexiones prácticas sobre La Relación Médico-Paciente. *Atención Primaria, 32*(10), 594–602.

Sánchez González, J. (2007). La relación médico-paciente. Algunos factores asociados que la afectan. *Revista CONAMED, 12*(1), 21–29.

Schufer, M. (1983). Algunos aspectos sociológicos de la relación médico-paciente. *Medicina y sociedad, 6*(4), 166–169.

Skirbekk, H., Middelthon, A., Hjortdahl, P., & Finset, A. (2011). Mandates of trust in the doctor-patient relationship. *Qualitative Health Research, 21*(9), 1182–1190.

Stern, M., Cotten, S., & Drentea, P. (2012). The separate spheres of online health: Gender, parenting, and online health information searching in the information age. *Journal of Family Issues, 33*(10), 1324–1350.

Thompson, A. G. H. (2007). The meaning of patient involvement and participation in health care consultations: A taxonomy. *Social Science and Medicine, 64*(6), 1297–1310.

Vidal y Benito, M. (2002). *Acerca de la buena comunicación en medicina* (1ra. edición). Buenos Aires: Instituto Universitario CEMIC.

Waisbord, S. (2015). Perspectivas críticas en comunicación y salud: ideas para investigaciones futuras. In M. Petracci (Ed.), *La salud en la trama comunicacional contemporánea* (pp. 141–151). Buenos Aires: Prometeo.

Wathen, C., & Harris, R. (2007). «I try to take care of it myself.» How rural women search for health information. *Qualitative Health Research, 17*(5), 639–651.

Wilkowska, W., & Ziefle, M. (2012). Privacy and data security in e-health: Requirements from the user's perspective. *Health Informatics Journal, 18*(3), 191–201.

Social disparities producing health inequities and shaping sickle cell disorder in Brazil

Clarice Santos Mota, Karl Atkin, Leny A. Trad and Ana Luisa A. Dias

ABSTRACT

Sickle cell disorder (SCD) is a severe recessive genetic condition manifesting in several complex forms. It is a cause of high mortality rates across the world, affecting predominantly non-white populations. This article aims to discuss how persistent social disparities and health inequalities in the Brazilian context can produce negative effects in lifelong conditions such as Sickle Cell Disorder. Appearing usually in the patient's first year of life, when not treated, SCD may lead to several life threatening complications and impact on a person's quality of life. In order to understand the link between health and social circumstances, it is important to consider the socio-economic transformation of Brazilian society over time, as well as cultural and historical aspects of the country. The concept of inequity will ground this analysis, facilitating an understanding of the process of producing an extra burden for people with SCD as a result of social disparities, including the existence of racism.

Introduction

The single Portuguese speaking country in Latin America, Brazil has 200,000,000 inhabitants and an immense landmass, divided into five regions, with great socio-cultural diversity and persistent social inequalities. Disproportionate distribution of wealth is an historically recognised problem in Brazil. Despite the huge variation of skin tones and other physical features of the Brazilian population, income inequality can be associated to lack of opportunities based on skin colour (Mitchell, 2010). This 'ethnoracial hierarchy' is not exclusively present in Brazil, but assumes different shades in Brazilian society, which can be related to a Latin American type of social stratification (Telles, Flores, & Urrea-Giraldo, 2015). Marked by 'race' mixture (mestizaje) and ethnic diversity, Latin American countries share a history of slavery and 'long-denied race-based inequalities' (Telles et al., 2015, p. 40).

For twenty years, Brazil experienced a military dictatorship, a period of intense political repression and violence by the state that lasted until 1985. The period of democratisation fostered an extensive debate and political mobilisation that resulted in the current Constitution, published in 1988, which legally guarantees the rights of Brazilians and the social protection of the state, and can be considered an advanced constitution with regard to citizenship and the state's commitment to health. The constitutional design sought to articulate universality and equity. In other words, it assured universal access to healthcare without distinctions regarding colour, class, faith, social or any other barriers. At the same time, it foresaw the need to implement targeted policies for social inclusion of vulnerable groups (Duarte, 2000; Fleury, 2011).

Currently, Brazil is facing a major political crisis resulting in a negative impact on the economy and living conditions. One of the first impacts of this crisis is the reduction of investment in social policies, the threat to democratic values and the extinction of equitable policies. In these circumstances health policies focused on minority populations are often the first to be abandoned due to neoliberal political strategies.

Equity is one of the main principles of the Brazilian National Health System (SUS), meaning that assuring full access to health care is crucial for a democratic society (Paim, 2006). In this sense, equity presupposes universality, since it is not possible to overcome inequities without ensuring that there is unrestricted access to services and decent health (Travassos, 1997). It also means that, in unequal contexts, universalist macrosocial public policies are not able to repair the inequities arising from the historical process of exclusion (Munanga, 2014). In other words, it is not a choice between one or the other principle, or to establish which is the most important, but indeed, to discuss the challenges of effecting equity. While the Brazilian Constitution legally provides the guarantee of access, equity seeks to provide social justice. It requires thinking about different health necessities of individuals and groups and the importance of policies of redistribution.

Inequities are unjust differences between groups and often emerge from unfair distribution of power, money and resources (Bhopal, 2014). Especially in multicultural societies, health policies must take into account cultural, social and economic factors that might influence health needs. Meeting the needs of different ethnic groups is challenging, but necessary to obtain improvements in health care. From the belief of inferiority of some groups, feelings of superiority may emerge, along with racist results. Racism is rarely explored in the understanding of health outcomes, although it can lead to socio-economic inequalities. Direct racism occurs by insults, harassment and mistreatment justified by feelings of superiority in relation to other groups, and is prohibited by law in most countries. Indirect racism is more subtle and results from decisions that favour some groups, which can be conceived as institutional racism when applied to organisations (Bhopal, 2014).

In this article we aim to discuss social disparities and health inequities in Brazil producing disadvantages for people with Sickle Cell Disorder, a condition more frequent among the non-white population. In order to understand how poorer life conditions and social inequalities produce negative health determinants it is crucial to examine social, cultural and historical variables. The historical background relating sickle cell disease to the 'black' population and slavery is very important when considering the social economic conditions of the people living with sickle cell disease today, mainly with a low socio-economic status and poor living conditions.

Racism is a result of historical social relations marked by slavery and reinforced by material deprivation and cultural-ideational structures such as negative stereotypes (Carter, 2000). In Brazil, the intersections between social class and racism have proved to be a determining factor in the accumulation of disadvantages among non-white groups. Santos (2009) emphasises the need to consider an analytical distinction between inequality of access and unequal treatment, to understand the racial inequality in Brazil.

There is no intention in discussing concepts of race neither considering race in the biological sense. Rather, to examine racism as unequal social relationships and the result of social forces, such as which reaffirm and develop hierarchies and inequalities (Ianni, 2004, p. 143). It is considered, furthermore, essential to recognise the peculiarities of social formation in the historical course of a given society (Omi & Howard, 1994), to analyse the social inequalities in their areas, as well as their effects. This process is especially required when trying to understand the complex dynamics of Brazilian society.

SCD: from a global scenario to the local context of Brazil

The S gene is carried by 7% of the population in the world and over 70% of all affected births occur in Africa (Ebrahim et al., 2010). Despite this, SCD is still considered the most neglected tropical disease worldwide (Ebrahim et al., 2010). It is estimated that there is a total amount of 300,000 births of children with SCD each year (Aygun & Odame, 2012; Dormandy et al., 2010) and projections for the future reveal that the frequency of SCD is expected to increase in sub-Saharan Africa and decrease in Eurasia, Americas and Arab-India by the year 2050 (Piel, Hay, Gupta, Weatherall, & Williams, 2013). Migration also contributes to the presence of this condition worldwide (Modell & Darlison, 2008), pointing towards the need of international effort to improve quality of life and assuring public health care for those facing this chronic disease.

Some studies show that the quality of life of SCD patients and their families is worse when compared to the general population and that the life expectancy of these people varies depending on the development of the country in which they reside (Dyson & Atkin, 2011). While some authors highlight a 'global burden of haemoglobin disorders' (Piel et al., 2013), mortality rates are disproportionately distributed over the world. In high-income countries the chance of surviving with a chronic disorder is much higher than in low-income countries, where children are at greater risk of dying before the age of 5 years (Modell & Darlison, 2008).

Historically, SCD was considered a 'childhood disease' that produced premature mortality, mostly due to infection, which can be directly related to social and environmental disadvantages (Platt et al., 1994). This pattern of mortality changed with early diagnosis, prophylactic penicillin and general improvements of socio-ecomomic conditions, which raised the life expectancy (Dennis-Antwi, Culley, Hiles, & Dyson, 2011). But still, in some parts of Africa, haemoglobin disorders contribute to 6.4% of mortality in children aged under 5 years, compared with 3.4% worldwide (Modell & Darlison, 2008).

The high mortality rates result not only from precarious living conditions, but also due to the difficulty accessing treatment, as well as the lack of research (Ebrahim et al., 2010). Full access to comprehensive health care can be lifesaving, since regular monitoring can prevent or minimise the complications of the disease. Nevertheless, Piel and collaborators (2013) will address the high costs of comprehensive health care, that usually involves a multi-professional team of health professionals.

All this leads us to reflect on the inequities in health and how they are differently expressed around the world. Considering SCD is present in many countries and has a global history, it is clear that there is a broader context that needs to be analysed. However, the Brazilian context is marked with the ambiguous character of its development model, which combines social achievements with remnants of poverty and inequalities.

Brazil is a developing country that has undergone major changes in recent years especially due to policies focused on redistribution of resources and poverty eradication. Between 1991 and 2008, the gross domestic product doubled and the Gini index fell from 0.637 to 0.547 and the poverty rate fell from 68% in 1970 to 31% in 2008. The living conditions also changed (Paim, Travassos, Almeida, Bahia, & Macinko, 2011). In 1970 only 33% of households had piped water and less than half had electricity. In 2007, the number of homes with piped water increased to 93% and almost all the houses have electricity. These changes affected the country's epidemiological profile raising the so-called 'diseases of modernity'. Cardiovascular diseases are the leading cause of death, followed by cancer and external causes, especially those resulting from traffic accidents and urban violence. Despite advances in living and health conditions, Brazil still suffers from inequalities (Paim et al., 2011), which mostly affects non-white populations (Heringer, 2002; Soares, 2008).

According to the census of 2010, from the Brazilian Institute of Geography and Statistics (IBGE), the so called 'black population' corresponds to more than half of the population (50.7%), a total of 190,732,694 people. It is worth noting that the term 'black population' is a social concept that corresponds to the total sum of all black and 'mixed-race' which are categories used by the national census. Therefore, a 'black person' in Brazil is anyone who claims to be black or of mixed race by self declaration in census surveys. The unification of these two categories was a political decision that occurred in 1996, to bring evidence towards statistical data regarding the social disadvantages of the non-white population in Brazil.

According to data from the Ministry of Health (SEPPIR) the 'black population' represents 67% of SUS (National Health System) users. In the last fifteen years, the country has reached some important goals to overcome extreme poverty and improve the living conditions of the most impoverished groups. Affirmative action policies such as quotas in education system, in addition to redistributive programs such as Bolsa Familia has been trying to overcome social inequalities. Especially income inequality between whites and non-whites has decreased from 2003 to 2010, even though it remains, as white workers still earn 1.8 times more than non-whites (Paixão & Rossetto, 2011).

Considering indicators of public health, studies on infant mortality indicated a reduction in their rates in the 70's and 90's, which, however, occurred unevenly between white and non-white children, with a 43% reduction rate for white children and 25% for non-white children. In 2006, the northeastern region had an infant mortality rate 24.2 times higher than that of the southern region, although this disparity has decreased (Paim et al., 2011).

Another equally suggestive indicator is the number of deaths of children under 5 years of age according to the cause of death, in which non-white children accounted for 55.6% of those who died due to acute diarrhoea (compared with 27.2% of white children), 49.0% who died from acute respiratory infection (37.5% of white children),

51.7% who died from malnutrition (28.9% of white children) and 54.4% of those who died of unknown causes from lack of medical care (24.7% of white children) (Paixão & Carvano, 2010).

In Brazil, the Ministry of Health estimated that there is one case of SCD per 1000 live births yearly (Cançado & Jesus, 2007). Screening is universally conducted, with 92% of newborns being screend, regardless of 'race'/colour (Amorim et al., 2010). In general, SCD is present in states and municipalities where there is a higher concentration of 'black population'. In Brazil the highest incidence is concentrated in Bahia, 1 per 650 live births (Cançado & Jesus, 2007). A higher incidence (1: 500) is registered in the state capital, the city of Salvador. A survey released by the Ministry of Health estimated a prevalence of 5.3% of Hb AS (sickle cell anaemia) in Bahia (Diniz Guedes, Barbosa, Tauil, & Magalhães 2009). Despite the high prevalence rates of sickle cell disease in Brazil, there are still very few studies focusing on the characterisation of the socio-demographic profile of SCD patients.

Recent studies show a reduction of up to 40% in SCD mortality with the use of Hydroxyurea in Brazil (Cançado, Lobo, & Ângulo, 2009). In November 2002, based on Decree 872, the Health Ministry approved the free use and distribution of HU for SCD patients. In the last fifteen years, the access to medication has shown a significant increase in quality of life for people suffering from the disorder, especially among the adult population (Silva & Shimauti, 2006). However, this same adult population born before the inclusion of the SCD in neonatal screening, which in general had a late diagnosis, presents a greater commitment to their health and quality of life.

In addition, one of the big challenges facing Brazil is the lack of reliable health data about this disease. This may itself be the result of a process that reveals a relative lack of political and academic interest in the subject and that certainly contributes towards the epidemiological and social invisibility of the disease and especially of the needs of those who face it. The enormous amount of research in biology and genetics, apart from the investment in clinical and pharmacological studies, has not been accompanied to the same extent by either epidemiological or sociological studies. Above all, there is a clear gap of systematic records of the number, spatial distribution, socio-demographic, morbidity and mortality profile of the people affected.

Due to the severity of the clinical manifestations of the disease, Brazil still faces high mortality rates. Such an outcome can happen to all types of SCD, however, patients with Sickle Cell Anaemia (Hb SS) commonly have the most severe clinical manifestations, and consequently, an increased risk of death (Fernandes, Januário, Cangussu, Macedo, & Viana, 2010). It was observed that 76% of deaths due to SCD occurred up to 29 years of age, with a concentration of 37% in children under nine, showing the severity of the disease (Loureiro & Rozenfeld, 2005). Considering that SCD is more frequent among the most impoverished, it is estimated that up to 25% of children do not reach 5 years of life. Perinatal mortality is also still very high in Brazil, ranging from 20% to 50% (Simoes, 2010).

In Brazil, it is observed, for example, that 85% of adults with SCD have a low level of education and those who manage to enter the labour market have jobs that require great physical effort, often incompatible with the course of the disease (Guimarães, Miranda, & Tavares, 2009). It is, therefore, a population with high social vulnerability, but the relationship between this issue and the course of the disease remains underexplored.

The daily routine of people with SCD involves a continuous process of care, both in the family context, as well as in the healthcare services, demanding rearrangements from the family in their routine, definition of responsibilities around the required care and availability of several types of resources. The routine of care, especially for children with SCD, interferes throughout the family system and often hinders the performance of other external functions, such as work, especially for mothers (Dias, 2013; Guimarães, 2009). Therefore, the disease can have dramatically different effects on employment opportunities, creating a cycle of impoverishment and commitment of family income, with a strong impact on the quality of life.

Absence from school may also be seen as a source of disadvantage that can limit social mobility. Frequent hospitalisation can lead to school absence and makes educational success even more challenging (Dias, Trad, & Castellanos, 2015). Mothers and young people with SCD usually have to negotiate and deal with some restrictive aspects of school routine and environment (Dyson, Atkin, Culley, Dyson, & Evans, 2011). It should also be considered that experiences of discrimination in school are a source of limitation, which can be associated with racism, although usually very subtly. Therefore, 'racism cannot be assumed to be absent on the basis of the lack of explicit references to the phenomenon, and consider the subtle ways that racism structures school experiences' (Dyson, Atkin, Culley, & Dyson, 2014, p. 2379). With historical roots, racism continues to inform relationships producing negative experiences both at the individual and collective level.

Furthermore, qualitative studies on experiences of people with SCD in Brazil show how they report recurrent feelings of being mistreated, neglected and discriminated against, inside the health services. These studies, based on the lived experiences of people with SCD, have consistently shown late diagnoses of the disease, lack of knowledge by the health professionals on how to manage the condition and symptoms and the search for care in different services. The suffering presented by these works are not only related to the condition per se, but as a result of the lack of knowledge, misconceptions and negative perceptions related to sickle cell disease, in some cases are present in the families, communities and also health services (Cordeiro, Ferreira, Santos, & Silva, 2013; Dias, 2013b; Xavier, 2011).

Can racism be taken as a form of social inequity affecting SCD?

Persistent health inequalities can also be interpreted as a result of social discrimination and political exclusion justified by negative conceptions around 'race', ethnicity, gender, sexual orientation, religion, and language. Patterns of advantage and disadvantage in society are not only socially constructed, but also (re-) produce inequalities in access, power, and status, thus marginalising some individuals. In this sense, the politics of equity represent the struggle for the human right to health (Hayden, 2012).

Reflections on how racism is present in our society makes it possible to understand the processes of production and reproduction of the disadvantages that certain individuals and population groups face and their negative impacts on health (Spencer, 2014). Although it is very complex to measure and demonstrate the effects of racism, it is important to consider in order to develop antiracist policies (Bhopal, 2014). In this section, we examine other variables besides material deprivation that may contribute to the understanding of social disadvantages faced by individuals with SCD. Thus, it is crucial to present historical aspects of Brazil, exploring social disparities as historically constructed social hierarchies, prejudices and discrimination.

Brazil was the Latin American country that imposed slavery on the largest number of individuals and the last Latin American country to end slavery. From 1538 to 1888, three hundred years of slavery marked Brazilian society and produced negative effects in its constitution as a nation. In post abolition years there was no effort towards social inclusion of this population, which means that racism needs to be considered as part of the cultural system available to powerful social agents who failed to initiate any strategies aimed at improving the material circumstances of the black population. Former slaves had no educational training and job places were most commonly occupied by skilled workers. At the end of the nineteenth century, there was a Brazilian government campaign to attract European immigrants to replace former slaves in the job market. Projections about the future of Brazil guided this policy, with the intention of 'improving' Brazilian 'racial stock', gradually 'whitening' future generations (Santos & Maio, 2004).

The failure to confront the racial issue in Brazil, historically covered up by the myth of racial democracy, ends up perpetuating inequalities. More than a myth, racial democracy should be seen as a historical political commitment by the Brazilian Government towards the establishment of a society with no inclusion of 'blacks' and other minorities (Guimarães, 2006). As a result, 'social inequalities in Brazil are tied to invisible mechanisms of racial discrimination that favour their expanded reproduction' (op cit, p. 280). Moreover, there was a political and ideological project of denying racism and concealing its consequences (op cit). Often, hidden dynamics of racism in society can produce shared experiences of misrecognition and non-recognition, rendering second-class citizenship.

The Brazilian system of racial classification is very complex. Characterised by a set of fluid categories, it combines skin colour with many other variables (Telles, 2002). Not only are physical traits, such as hair, lips and nose considered to be variables, but also social position (Guimarães, 2012). It is also crucial to consider how these categories change over time and a historical sight must be taken in order to fully understand these issues. More recently, a race-based identity is becoming stronger, associated with the involvement with 'black' activists' movements, with the emergence of a 'black' middle class and with political mobilisation (Kay, Mitchell, & White, 2015; Maio & Monteiro, 2005).

Considering racism as an obstacle to social mobility, it is possible to examine how it operates in a Brazilian context. First, as a cultural system, in which non-whites are perceived in a depreciatory way, commonly related to criminal violence, poverty, ignorance etc. These perceptions negatively affect the labour market and family income as a consequence. Second, there are indicators of social vulnerability that affects mostly non-white families, such as poor housing conditions, neighbourhoods with lower quality of public services as well as high rates of violence, including police violence and homicides. These families usually cannot afford private schools, which makes it harder to enter universities, negatively affecting social mobility.

Therefore, admitting that there is a structural dimension that goes beyond interpersonal relations, and that racial inequalities in Brazil are not just a matter of material deprivation, means recognising the complexity of this phenomenon. Sickle cell disorder is not immune to this process, since 'experiences of racial harassment and discrimination, and perceptions of living in a discriminatory society, contribute to ethnic inequalities in health' (Nazroo, Williams, Marmot, & Wilkinson, 2006, p. 260).

According to Bediako and Moffitt (2011), studies that explore the social meanings and attitudes around SCD may have important implications in clinical care. In the UK, SCD became associated with the politics of 'race' rather than the disadvantage associated with having a long term condition, which might create disabling consequences (Berghs, Atkin, Graham, Hatton, & Thomas, 2016). The policy neglect of SCD, could be attributed to institutionalised racism, in which the needs of ethnic minority groups were ignored or misrepresented (Kalckman, Santos, Batista, & Cruz, 2007; Lopez, 2012; Silvério, 2002). While relevant, such an analysis tends to ignore the broader social disparities associated with having a long term condition.

Race ideas and stereotypes may emerge from negative perceptions carried out in society that potentially influence how people see SCD (Bediako & Moffitt, 2011; Tapper, 1999; Wailoo, 1997, 2001). For example, the association with drug use, has led health professionals to deny pain medication, labelling people with SCD as being addicted to painkillers (Atkin & Anionwu, 2010; Rouse, 2004). Other studies also claim that SCD association with race has led to poor health services, where racism is one of the explanatory factors for the low priority that haemoglobinopathies have in public health care (Cordeiro and Ferreira, 2009; Dyson & Atkin, 2011).

In the Brazilian context, where people with sickle cell disorder are predominately blacks, it is worth analysing how social disadvantages can add an extra burden to the disease experience. It is essential to discuss the convergence between social disparities and racism, when making sense of SCD. It is possible that poverty will interact with depreciative representations produced by racism to create negative consequences for health outcomes. Nevertheless, this association is not simple to prove, since the relationship among health inequalities and racism is a complex and dynamic one (Carter, 2000). Further studies are required, in order to examine more carefully the interaction between racism and material deprivation as determinants of health inequalities (Chor & Lima, 2005; Kabad, Bastos, & Santos, 2012; Chor, 2013).

In order to measure these inequalities, it is not only a question of observing the discrepancy in mortality patterns, but also considering aspects related to quality of life. Apart from the clinical vulnerability caused by the very symptoms of the disease, social vulnerability interacting with racism can set up a process of disadvantage overlays. Such disadvantages, when not causing premature death, are responsible for consequences that could be prevented with health provision and good living conditions.

There are few studies in Brazil that analyse the impact of racism in the care offered to people with SCD. Considering the potential interactions of income, gender and skin colour in understanding how appropriate care is accessed, one's relationship to health service provision represent social relationships and therefore reproduce social hierarchies and existing forms of discrimination. Especially if we consider that, in general, the health policies are devised and planned by hegemonic sectors of society, which often disregard the needs of minorities (Bhopal, 2007).

Moreover, the disabling consequences of chronic, life long conditions such as SCD are also produced by various structural disadvantage that people might face. Nonetheless, to make sense of these structures, we need to treat them as analytically distinct and in particular explore material circumstances independently from the ideas that generate discriminatory practices such as racism. It is equally important to distinguish between the structures of discrimination and the human actions, which can reinforce them. Focusing on human actions, rather than the inevitably of structural determinism, creates the possibility of transformative action, which may (or may not) transform those structures. To be successful, such transformative action, requires reflexive engagement in which analytical distinctions are understood, as the basis of knowing insight, in which specific consequences can be attributed to specific interventions (Carter, 2000).

Final considerations

In the 25 years since the World Health Organization identified SCD as a relevant problem of public health significance, 'the majority of children in resource-poor countries have not benefited from the many advances in treatment and care' (Ebrahim et al., 2010). Although it is a serious disease with complex and varied manifestations, the course of SCD could be improved by better access to full, continuous and humanised care.

Frequently, in periods of economic crisis like the one Brazil faces today, minorities are most penalised not only because of intensification of poverty, but also as a consequence of the extinction of social policies focused on (re-) distribution of wealth and power. Those are the times in which the struggle for equity as social justice needs to be intensified, while individuals and groups need to raise their attention to the risk of losing constitutional rights.

Equity is especially relevant to SCD policies because, despite advances in treatment, in many countries people still don't have full access to it. It is possible that in some contexts, SCD received less public and professional support compared with other less prevalent diseases, including research funding.

To reduce inequalities and promote equity, health policies should address the needs of groups (Bhopal, 2014). In the Brazilian Universal Health System, social participation is another principle that establishes mechanisms of dialogue and control of society. In the history of health policies for SCD in Brazil, the role of health activism was, and still is, very important. Most achievements are results of pressure from organised social movements, specifically formed by people suffering from the condition and their families. The social movement of people and families with SCD is an example of mobilisation and struggle for rights to health. This is a good example of how ethnic minorities have conquered significant political achievements and developed resilience despite adversity (Anionwu & Atkin, 2001; Dias, 2013).

The discussion about racism presented here is grounded in the fact that the 'race'/ colour should not be taken in the biological sense. Nevertheless, it must be considered that 'racial bias adversely affects the availability of resources not only for research and the delivery of care, but also for the improvement of that care' (Smith, Oyeku, Homer, & Zuckerman, 2006, p. 1767). It is crucial to examine the results of social disparities in the production of health inequities, and the necessity of redistributive policies aimed at the promotion of equity as social justice. Although explained by historical roots, the continuation of these inequalities concerns and encourages us to think of the challenges for the achievement of a just society.

By bringing the issue of social inequalities linked to a chronic disease such as SCD, an attempt was made to consider the unique aspects of the Brazilian social context. Providing elements to understand to what extent the socio-economic disparities and shared experiences of racial harrassment can be a source of vulnerability. Other researchers have already discussed this correlation, but Bediako, Lavender, and Yasin (2007) points to the need for more studies to explore the different socio-cultural factors that interfere with the course of the disease. Not only macro-economic variables, such as income and social status, but also aspects related to the dynamics of the family, social support, and personal experience should be investigated. Regarding the absence of such studies, he warns: 'until sociocultural influences such as racial identity are explicitly investigated and well understood, treatment strategies for sickle cell pain will continue to have a one-dimensional pathophysiological focus' (op cit, 2007, p. 434).

Although the correlation between life and health conditions is relevant to any form of disease, there are specific aspects relevant to SCD, given its chronic condition. That is, one cannot deny that impoverishment affects any chronic disease, but in the case of a condition whose symptoms appear already in the first year of life, inequities can greatly affect the entire course of the patient's life. All too often, adults at a productive working age find themselves unable to work due to the degree of sequelae. There is then the broader impact to the adults' quality of life. It is, therefore, urgent to take into account in future research the weight that racism brings to the experience with illness, as it often exceeds even the weight of the disease itself (Atkin & Ahmad, 2001).

It is also crucial to invest in training professionals at primary healthcare centres to identify risks and signs of complications. Neonatal screening, prophylactic penicillin, immunisation and self care strategies are simple, but necessary, interventions (Fernandes et al., 2010). In addition, the articulation of the primary care network with hospital services and haematologist clinics remains a goal to be achieved.

It can be concluded that a greater effort to understand Latin American countries and their cultural singularities can bring new insights to health determinants and patterns of disease. Considering the similarities between these emerging economies, new partnerships can render joint efforts towards different ways of thinking, coping and living with Sickle Cell Disorder.

Disclosure statement

No potential conflict of interest was reported by the authors.

Funding

This work was supported by Conselho Nacional de Desenvolvimento Científico e Tecnológico.

References

Amorim, T., Pimentel, H., Fontes, M. I. M. M., Purificação, A., Lessa, P., & Boa-Sorte, N. (2010). Avaliação do programa de triagem neonatal da Bahia entre 2007 e 2009–as lições da doença falciforme. *Gazeta Médica da Bahia*, 3, 10–13.

Anionwu, E., & Atkin, K. (2001). *The politics of sickle cell and Thalassaemia*. Buckingham: Open University Press.

Atkin, K., & Ahmad, W. I. U. (2001). Living a 'normal' life: Young people coping with thalassaemia major or sickle cell disorder. *Social Science & Medicine*, 53(5), 615–626. doi:10.1016/S0277-9536(00)00364-6

Atkin, K., & Anionwu, E. (2010). *The social consequences of sickle cell and Thalassaemia: Improving the quality of support*. London: Race Equality Foundation.

Aygun, B., & Odame, I. (2012). A global perspective on sickle cell disease. *Pediatric, Blood and Cancer, 59*, 386–390.

Bediako, S. M., Lavender, A. R., & Yasin, Z. (2007). Racial centrality and health care use among African American adults with sickle cell disease. *Journal of Black Psychology, 33*(4), 422–438.

Bediako, S. M., & Moffitt, K. (2011). Race and social attitudes about sickle cell disease. *Ethnicity & Health, 16*(4–5), 423–429. doi:10.1080/13557858.2011.552712

Berghs, M., Atkin, K., Graham, H., Hatton, C., & Thomas, C. (2016). Implications for public health research of models and theories of disability: A scoping review and evidence synthesis. *Public Health Research, 4*(8), 1–166.

Bhopal, R. S. (2007). *Ethnicity, race, and health in multicultural societies: Foundations for better epidemiology, public health, and health care.* Oxford: Oxford University Press.

Bhopal, R. S. (2014). *Migration, ethnicity, race, and health in multicultural societies.* Oxford: Oxford University Press.

Cançado, R. D., & Jesus, J. A. (2007). A doença falciforme no Brasil. *Revista Brasileira de Hematologia e Hemoterapia*, São José do Rio Preto, *29*(3), 203–206.

Cançado, R. D., Lobo, C., & Ângulo, I. L. (2009). Protocolo clínico e diretrizes terapêuticas para uso de hidroxiureia na doença falciforme. *Revista Brasileira de Hematologia e Hemoterapia, 31*(5), 361–366.

Carter, B. (2000). *Racism and realism: Concepts of race in sociological research.* London: Routledge.

Chor, D. (2013). Health inequalities in Brazil: Race matters. *Cadernos de Saúde Pública, 29*(7), 1272–1275 . doi:10.1590/S0102-311X201300070000

Chor, D., & Lima, C. R. D. A. (2005). Epidemiologic aspects of racial inequalities in health in Brazil. *Cadernos de Saúde Pública, 21*(5), 1586–1594. doi:10.1590/S0102-311X2005000500033

Cordeiro, R. C., & Ferreira, S. L. (2009). Discriminação racial e de gênero em discursos de mulheres negras com anemia falciforme [Racial and gender discrimination on the discourses of black women with sickle cell anemia]. *Escola Anna Nery* [online], *13*(2), 352–358.

Cordeiro, R. C., Ferreira, S. L., Santos, F. C., & Silva, L. S. (2013). Itinerários terapêuticos de pessoas com anemia falciforme face às crises dolorosas. *Revista Enfermagem UERJ, 2*, 179–184.

Dennis-Antwi, J. A., Culley, L., Hiles, D., & Dyson, S. M. (2011). "I can die today, I can die tomorrow": Lay perceptions of sickle cell disease in Kumasi, Ghana at a point of transition. *Ethnicity and Health, 16*(4-5), 465–481.

Dias, A. L. (2013). Da invisibilidade ao reconhecimento: A importância da Associação Baiana das Pessoas com Doença Falciforme na trajetória dos(as) associados(as) e seus familiares. In S. L. Ferreira & R. C. Cordeiro (Eds.) (organizadoras), *Qualidade de vida e cuidados às pessoas com doença falciforme* (pp. 95–112). Salvador: EDUFBA.

Dias, A. L. A. (2013b). *A (re)construção do caminhar: itinerário terapêutico de pessoas com doença falciforme com histórico de úlcera de perna (Dissertação de mestrado).* Universidade Federal da Bahia, Instituto de Saude Coletiva, Salvador.

Dias, A. L. A., Trad, L. A. B., & Castellanos, M. E. (2015). Infância e Adolescência com Doença Falciforme: uma juventude diferenciada In: Cronicidade: 263 p.

Diniz, D., Guedes, C., Barbosa, L., Tauil, P. L., & Magalhães, I. (2009). Prevalência do traço e da anemia falciforme em recém-nascidos do Distrito Federal, Brasil, 2004 a 2006. *Cad. Saúde Pública, Rio de Janeiro, 25*, 188–194.

Dormandy, E., Gulliford, M., Bryan, S., Roberts, T. E., Calnan, M., Atkin, K., & Johnston, T. A. (2010). Effectiveness of earlier antenatal screening for sickle cell disease and thalassaemia in primary care: Cluster randomised trial. *British Medical Journal, 341*, c5132, 1–10.

Duarte, C. M. R. (2000). Eqüidade na legislação: um princípio do sistema. *Ciência e Saúde Coletiva, 5*(2), 443–463.

Dyson, S., & Atkin, K. (2011). Sickle cell and Thalassaemia: Global public health issues come of age. In S. Dyson & K. Atkin (Eds.), *Genetics and global public health* (pp. 1–13). London: Routledge.

Dyson, S., Atkin, K., Culley, L., & Dyson, S. (2014). Critical realism, agency and sickle cell: Case studies of young people with sickle cell disorder at school. *Ethnic and Racial Studies, 37*(13), 2379–2398.

Dyson, S. M., Atkin, K., Culley, L. A., Dyson, S. E., & Evans, H. (2011). Sickle cell, habitual dys-positions and fragile dispositions: Young people with sickle cell at school. *Sociology of Health & Illness*, 33(3), 465–483.

Ebrahim, S. H., Khoja, T. A. M., Elachola, H., Atrash, H. K., Memish, Z., & Johnson, A. (2010). Children who come and go. The state of sickle cell disease in resource-poor countries. *American Journal of Preventive Medicine*, 38(4S), S568–S570.

Fernandes, A. P. P. C., Januário, J. N., Cangussu, C. B., Macedo, D. L. D., & Viana, M. B. (2010). Mortality of children with sickle cell disease: A population study. *Jornal de Pediatria*, 86(4), 279–284.

Fleury, S. (2011). Unfair inequalities: The health care counter right. *Psicologia & Sociedade*, 23 (SPE), 45–52.

Guimarães, A. S. A. (2006). Depois da democracia racial [After racial democracy]. *Tempo Social*, 18 (2), 269–287. doi:10.1590/S0103-20702006000200014

Guimarães, A. S. A. (2009). *Racismo e Antirracismo no Brasil*. São Paulo: Editora 34.

Guimarães, A. S. A. (2012). The Brazilian system of racial classification. *Ethnic and Racial Studies*, 35(7), 1157–1162. doi:10.1080/01419870.2011.632022

Guimarães, T. M. R., Miranda, W. L., & Tavares, M. M. F. (2009). O cotidiano das famílias de crianças e adolescentes portadores de anemia falciforme. *Revista Brasileira de Hematologia e Hemoterapia*, São Paulo, 31(1), 9–14.

Hayden, P. (2012). The human right to health and the struggle for recognition. *Review of International Studies*, 38(03), 569–588.

Heringer, R. (2002). Desigualdades raciais no Brasil: síntese de indicadores e desafios no campo das políticas públicas [Racial inequalities in Brazil: A synthesis of social indicators and challenges for public policies]. *Cadernos de Saúde Pública*, 18(Suppl.), S57–S65. doi:10.1590/S0102-311X2002000700007

Ianni, O. (2004). A Questão Social. In *Octavio Ianni - Pensamento Social no Brasil*. Bauru, SP: EDUSC.

Kabad, J. F., Bastos, J. L., & Santos, R. V. (2012). Raça, cor e etnia em estudos epidemiológicos sobre populações brasileiras: revisão sistemática na base PubMed [Race, color and ethnicity in epidemiologic studies carried out with Brazilian populations: Systematic review on the PubMed database]. *Physis: Revista de Saúde Coletiva*, 22(3), 895–918 . doi:10.1590/S0103-73312012000300004

Kalckman, S., Santos, C. G., Batista, L. E., & Cruz, V. M. (2007). Racismo institucional: um desafio pra a equidade no SUS? *Saúde e Sociedade*, 16(2), 146–155.

Kay, K., Mitchell, G., & White, I. K. (2015). Framing race and class in Brazil: Afro-Brazilian support for racial versus class policy. *Politics, Groups, and Identities*, 3(2), 222–238.

Lopez, L. C. (2012). O conceito de racismo institucional: Aplicações no campo da saúde. *Interface - Comunicação, Saúde, Educação* [online], 16(40), 121–134.

Loureiro, M. M., & Rozenfeld, S. (2005). Epidemiologia de internações por Doença Falciforme no Brasil. *Revista de Saúde Pública*, Ano 39(6), 943–949.

Maio, M., & Monteiro, S. (2005). Tempos de racialização: o caso da 'saúde da população negra' no Brasil [In times of racialization: The case of the 'health of the black population' in Brazil]. *História, Ciências, Saúde-Manguinhos*, Rio de Janeiro, 12(2), 419–446 . doi:10.1590/S0104-59702005000200010

Mitchell, G. L. (2010). Racism and Brazilian democracy: Two sides of the same coin? *Ethnic and Racial Studies*, 33(10), 1776–1796.

Modell, B., & Darlison, M. (2008). Global epidemiology of haemoglobin disorders and derived service indicators. *Bulletin of the World Health Organization*, 86(6), 480–487.

Munanga, K. (2014). A questão da diversidade e da política de reconhecimento das diferenças. *Revista Crítica e Sociedade*, 4(1), 34–45.

Nazroo, J. Y., & Williams, D. R. (2006). The social determination of ethnic/racial inequalities in health. In: M. G. Marmot & R. G. Wilkinson (Eds.), *Social determinants of health*. New York, NY: Oxford University Press.

Omi, M., & Howard, W. (1994). *Racial formation in the United States: From the 1960s to the1990s* (2nd ed.). New York and London: Routledge.

Paim, J. S. (2006). Equidade e Reforma em Sistemas de Serviços de Saúde: o caso do SUS. *Saúde e Sociedade, 15*(2), 34–46.

Paim, J., Travassos, C., Almeida, C., Bahia, L., & Macinko, J. (2011). The Brazilian health system: History, advances, and challenges, health in Brazil 1. *The Lancet, 377*, 1778–1797. doi:10.1016/S0140-6736(11)60054-8

Paixão, M., & Carvano, L. M. (2010). Censo e Demografia. A variável cor ou raça no interior dos sistemas censitários brasileiros. In L. E Sansone & O. A. Pinho (Eds.), *Raça: Novas perspectivas antropológicas*. Salvador: Associação Brasileira de Antropologia. Edufba, 2ª edição rev.

Paixão, M., & Rossetto, I. (2011). Balanço dos oito anos do Governo Lula sobre as assimetrias de cor ou raça. *Tempo em Curso, 3*(2), 1–13.

Piel, F. B., Hay, S. I., Gupta, S., Weatherall, D. J., & Williams, T. N. (2013). Global burden of sickle cell anaemia in children under five, 2010–2050: Modelling based on demographics, excess mortality, and interventions. *PLoS Medicine, 10*(7), e1001484. doi:10.1371/journal.pmed.1001484

Platt, O. S., Brambilla, D. J., Rosse, W. F., Milner, P. F., Castro, O., Steinberg, M. H., & Klug, P. P. (1994). Mortality in sickle cell disease--life expectancy and risk factors for early death. *New England Journal of Medicine, 330*(23), 1639–1644.

Rouse, C. M. (2004). Paradigms and politics: Shaping health care access for sickle cell patients through the discursive regimes of biomedicine. *Culture, Medicine and Psychiatry, 28*(3), 369–399.

Santos, J. A. F. (2009). A interação estrutural entre a desigualdade de raça e de gênero no Brasil. *Revista Brasileira de Ciências Sociais* [online], *24*(70), 37–60. [cited 2016-10-27]

Santos, R. V., & Maio, M. C. (2004). Qual" retrato do Brasil"? Raça, biologia, identidades e política na era da genômica. *Mana, 10*(1), 61–95.

Silva, M. C., & Shimauti, E. L. T. (2006). Eficácia e toxicidade da hidroxiuréia em crianças com anemia falciforme. *Revista Brasileira de Hematologia e Hemoterapia*, São José do Rio Preto, *28*(2), 144–148.

Silvério, V. R. (2002). Ação afirmativa e o combate ao racismo institucional no Brasil [Affirmative action and the fight against institutional racism in Brazil]. *Cadernos de Pesquisa, 10*(117), 219–246. doi:10.1590/S0100-15742002000300012

Simoes, B. P. (2010). Consenso brasileiro em transplante de células-tronco hematopoéticas: Comitê de hemoglobinopatias. *Revista Brasileira de Hematologia e Hemoterapia* [online], *32*(suppl.1), 46–53.

Smith, L. A., Oyeku, S. O., Homer, C., & Zuckerman, B. (2006). Sickle cell disease: A question of equity and quality. *Pediatrics, 117*(5), 1763–1770.

Soares, S. (2008). A Demografia da Cor: A Composição da População Brasileira de 1890 a 2007. In M Theodoro, L. Jaccoud, R. Osório, & S. Soares (Eds.), *As políticas públicas e a desigualdade racial no Brasil: 120 anos após a abolição* (pp. 97–117). Brasília: Ipea.

Spencer, S. (2014). *Race and ethnicity: Culture, identity and representation*. New York: Routledge.

Tapper, M. (1999). *In the blood – sickle cell anemia and the politics of race*. Philadelphia: University of Pennsylvania Press, 163 p.

Telles, E. E. (2002). Racial ambiguity among the Brazilian population. *Ethnic and Racial Studies, 25*(3), 415–441.

Telles, E., Flores, R. D., & Urrea-Giraldo, F. (2015). Pigmentocracies: Educational inequality, skin color and census ethnoracial identification in eight Latin American countries. *Research in Social Stratification and Mobility, 40*, 39–58.

Travassos, C. (1997). Eqüidade e o Sistema Único de Saúde: uma contribuição para debate. *Cadernos de Saúde Pública, 13*(2), 325–330.

Wailoo, K. (1997). Detecting 'negro blood': Black and white identities and the reconstruction of sickle cell anemia. In Keith Wailoo (Ed.), *Drawing blood: Technology and disease identity in twentieth century america* (pp. 134–161). Baltimore: The Johns Hopkins University Press.

Wailoo, K. (2001). *Dying in the city of the blues: Sickle cell anemia and the politics of race and health*. Chapel Hill: The University of North Carolina Press.

Xavier, A. S. G. (2011). *Experiências reprodutivas de mulheres com anemia falciforme (Dissertação)*. Salvador: Universidade Federal da Bahia, Escola de Enfermagem.

Socio/Ethno-epidemiologies: proposals and possibilities from the Latin American production

Anahi Sy

ABSTRACT

This article presents an approach to understanding health that acquires an original and autonomous development across different Latin American countries, despite being the result of reading and analysing national and international theoretical contributions from social sciences. The proposal seeks to integrate the epidemiologic perspective with those from the social sciences, sociology, and medical anthropology in particular, raising the need to place health problems in their socio-historic, cultural, political and economic context. From this framework, such aspects must be treated not only as epidemiological variables but, above all, as sociocultural and bio-ecological processes. It suggests to conceptually work from a perspective that investigates health-disease as a social process, an area of life in which most of the meanings, representations and practices that allow the reproduction of daily life are articulated. For that, we place the contributions in the field of Collective Health, present the main criticisms and limitations that have been raised to modern epidemiology and, from there, we develop theoretic-methodological proposals of ethno-epidemiology and sociocultural epidemiology directing the analysis towards the development of a superseding episteme.

Introduction

The current state of knowledge and development of research in epidemiology has posed serious difficulties in responding to health problems at the population level. Although more sophisticated methodologies and analytical techniques are available, the generated discussions and criticisms, not only within the field but also from external sources, are becoming more frequent. This raises the need to develop a way of approaching health and illness in current society from a superseding perspective.

Starting from the criticisms and limitations posed to modern epidemiology, this article proposes an innovative field of knowledge that is developing autonomously in the Latin American setting. This is known as 'sociocultural epidemiology' or 'ethno-epidemiology' and will be generically labelled here as *socio/ethno-epidemiologies*. It is positioned in the field of Collective Health, and its focus goes beyond public health, community medicine, and preventive and social medicine (see Almeida Filho & Silva Paim, 1999; Frenk, 1992; Liborio, 2013; Paim, 1992, 2011; Sousa Campos, 2000).

Collective Health, as it has been built since 1970, results from two main sources: the criticism of the different health reform projects and movements occurred in capitalist countries and; the theoretic-epistemological elaboration and scientific production articulated in social practices. In Latin America, the theoretical work produced in the last forty years has redefined the field of public health-differentiating it from the way in which it has been traditionally conceived in Europe and the United States (Paim, 1992). Collective Health has been defined as a field of thought and scope of practices (Almeida Filho & Silva Paim, 1999) produced in, and from, Latin America, with the conviction that, to understand what happens in our countries, the elaborations must be local (Testa, 1992; Testa y Paim, 2010) – since there are many examples of unsuccessful imported models of care.

Thus, the designation of Collective Health acquires a much broader connotation than that of Public Health, which includes social medicine – a trend of thought that emerged as a criticism of the latter one–and reflects the development of social sciences in the field of health (Paim, 1992). Its theoretic-epistemological framework refers to an interdisciplinary field and not properly to a scientific discipline or medical specialty (Almeida Filho & Silva Paim, 1999). It focuses on the construction of new theories, approaches and methods in epidemiology and health planning, incorporating concrete investigations that apply the methodology and theories of social sciences in the field of health. From that theoretic-methodological effort, new modalities have emerged of interdisciplinary qualitative and quantitative approaches that delimit new objects of knowledge and intervention. Examples of these include the so-called 'Sociocultural Epidemiology' and the 'Ethno-epidemiology', which are studied in this article.

Criticisms of modern epidemiology

Criticisms about modern epidemiology have become increasingly frequent in Latin America (Almeida Filho, 1992a, 1992b, 2000, 2007; Álvarez Hernández, 2008; Barata & Barreto, 1996; Barreto, 1998; Breilh, 1995, 1997; Diez Roux, 2004, 2007; Haro, 2010; Silva Ayçaguer, 1997, 2005; Sy, 2009), as in the rest of the world, especially in North America (Krieger, 1994; Long, 1993; McMichael, 1995, 1999; Pearce, 1996, 2007, 2008; Rothman, 2007; Shy, 1997; Sterne and Smith, 2001; Susser & Susser, 1996a, 1996b; Taubes & Mann, 1995). Though this article will not expand on this topic, it is necessary to give an account of these criticisms in order to better understand the superseding potential of socio/ethno-epidemiology.

An interview by Taubes and Mann (1995), published in *Science* is just one of the works that, arguably, has had more repercussion within and outside the epidemiological field. The work titled 'Epidemiology faces its limits'[1] gathers the opinions of prominent epidemiologists and biostatisticians regarding some fundamental methodological problems that epidemiology has not been able to overcome. The main issues are, on the one hand, that epidemiology, through the publication of uncertain research results and, on occasions, contradictory research result, generates anxiety among the public, false expectations and disbelief. On the other hand, the nature of epidemiological research methods and design can be weak. These matters are not new, both before and after this interview, the questions about such issues were present and still are (Álvarez Hernández, 2008). In the Latin American setting, the Brazilian epidemiologist, Maurício Barreto (1998) published 'For an epidemiology of collective health',[2] where he discusses that the challenge of modern epidemiology is to solve the problems that affect the health of populations. He proposes to systematize criticisms to delineate an epidemiology that contributes to the field of 'collective health'. Barreto (1998) identifies a crisis in the dominant paradigm; in its capacity of theoretical elaboration; for breaking away from its historical commitment; and in relation to the practice of public health and its explanatory capabilities, a crisis of conflicting results generated by different studies on the same topic.

In this sense, the Argentine epidemiologist based in the US, Ana Diez Roux (2004) warns about the fragmentation of the field because of the different 'types' of epidemiology: 'social' epidemiology, epidemiology of 'risk factors' and 'genetic' epidemiology, each of them with its own literature. Furthermore, in a series of editorials in *Collective Health* [3] magazine, she discusses some of the criticisms with Brazilian epidemiologist Naomar de Almedida Filho. Diez Roux (2007) wrote 'For an epidemiology with more numbers',[4] which is an answer to the provocation by Almeida Filho's book 'Epidemiology without numbers',[5] published in 1992. In her editorial, Diez Roux highlights as criticism of modern epidemiology, its growing methodological sophistication, which has resulted in an individualisation of problems and the biologisation of its study subject, which delimits the determinants of health exclusively at the level of biological characteristics. This concern is centred on the emphasis of biological measurement in epidemiology, with distrust over the utility or importance to health of the so-called 'soft' social or cultural variables. The most extreme expression of this process is the genetic determinism, increasingly discredited among geneticists themselves (Diez Roux, 2007).

In response, Almeida Filho (2007) wrote 'for an epidemiology with (more than) numbers: how to overcome the false quantitative and qualitative opposition'.[6] In it, Almeida Filho (2007) points out that the 'qualitative vs quantitative' opposition is unhelpful when it comes to establishing agreements to produce knowledge regarding concrete problems of nature, culture, society and history regarding health. He proposes a typology of studies methodologically integrated composed by three types:

> Combinations, strategies that articulate in the area of logistics, techniques of another methodological registry; Methodological compounds, mixed strategies where, for example, one can have two stages in one study; Methodological complexes, which are methodological hybrids.

What is clear, here, is that the focus is on the methodologic – difficulty lays in an epidemiology whose mathematization is abstracted from dimensions which, for many, cannot be quantified.

On this matter, the Mexican epidemiologist Gerardo Álvarez Hernández (2008) raises two core issues about the conceptualisation of modern epidemiology. Firstly, its propensity to the exclusive use of statistics as validation method and, secondly, the weakness of the theoretical constructs used to substantiate study methods. Both characteristics can be explained by the biologicist and individualist focus rooted in the positivist paradigm used by modern epidemiology to approach health problems. (Álvarez, 2008).

Likewise, it is observed that most epidemiological studies generally use different pre-established variables such as sex, age, social stratification, or occupational level, among others, without a reflection on the relevance of evaluating them in a particular population. The tendency is to group or classify the population according parameters that do not account for its ethnic or cultural specificity. These variables acquire similar values in all the poor or marginal sectors of the developing countries. Thus, the outcomes of such studies only contribute circular explanations of a general nature that do not aim to explain the problem due to particular socio-political, economic, cultural and historical characteristics and conditions (Sy, 2009). As pointed out by Bourdieu, Chamboredon, and Passeron (2008), when relying on factors that are transhistoric and transcultural, one runs the risk of assuming that what needs an explanation has been explained. This approach leaves unexplained what determines the historical specificity or cultural originality of the problem one seeks to understand.

It is argued that 'globalization' has tended to homogenise health problems and populations. This might be the case with epidemiology, though discussions regarding the 'epidemiological transition' would problematise it. However, in social and cultural terms, the reality in Latin America is characterised by the ethnic, racial, sexual, gender, historical, economic, environmental, and climate diversities, among others. These coexist and overlap in a more or less coherent or contradictory manner. The inequalities are not homogenous, and that is the limit to statistical standardisation or generalisation. It is true that one can measure degrees of inequality defined a priori, or independently of the populations where they will be applied. Nevertheless, it is also true that inequality is not expressed in the same way in a *villa miseria* (shanty town) than in a rural area. Even in the latter, it is not the same amongst indigenous or peasant populations (Sy, 2009, 2013). It is also not the same if each of these sectors are placed in Argentina, Mexico, or Brazil. There is diversity in inequality, and the invisibilization of cultures or ethnicities, languages, of habits and habitats, of socio-historical trajectories, environmental and economic diversities of the populations, which allow a better understanding of the current situation, has been one of the main difficulties in the strategies to improve health situations. This invisibilization has led to interventions being standardised.

As argued by Almeida Filho (1992b), though in most Latin American countries the models and policies of health care have been redefined, the health conditions of the populations have not been improved in the same manner. The explanations for this apparent paradox can be found in the inadequate conceptual basis of planning, as well as the organisation and administration of health services that rely almost exclusively on a conventional epidemiological perspective which does not take into account the historical and sociocultural nature of health problems.

Even the World Health Organization's Commission on Social Determinants of Health (CSDH) has pointed out that, though many health problems can be attributed to the socioeconomic conditions of people, the design and execution of health policies have been centred on the treatment of illnesses. Such approach does not consider 'the causes of the causes', which can, undoubtedly, be identified in the social context. It is acknowledged that there is enough scientific evidence–mostly from developed countries–to carry out concrete actions to reduce inequities in health, though there is not a systematic effort to implement them. The CSDH also points out that a final understanding of the role played by social and cultural factors in the epidemiological profile of the population seems unlikely under the biomedical approach of modern epidemiology. Thus, the Commission recommended the exploration of innovative methodologies that are susceptible to the application in human populations (Commission on Social Determinants of Health, WHO, 2005).

One socio/ethno-epidemiology, or many?

In the Latin American setting, like others, social epidemiology is not homogenous, nor exempt from discussions amongst the different actors. It is a field that is still being defined and redefined both theoretically and empirically.

To talk about socio-epidemiology, social or sociocultural epidemiology means to take a position regarding those who, like Almeida-Filho (2000), argue that it is a 'scandalous redundancy' (p. 137) since the social-collective is already contained in the designative *demos*, as in the object of knowledge of epidemiological science. Although it also refers to a 'successful redundancy' (p. 155) in stating that it was not expected that the difficulty of epidemiology would fall precisely in its ability to address the social. Thus, this author, will start from a criticism, not only to modern epidemiology–as one previously developed– but also to Latin American social medicine. Particularly, to the proposal by Laurell (1983), raising the difficulty of understanding the health-disease process from the category of 'work process', or the one proposed by Breilh and Granda (1986) of 'social reproduction'. This would result in a reduction of the social complexity to only one dimension of life and highlights the need of considering other dimensions in the process, such as the symbolic and the everyday life (Almeida Filho, 1993).

Betancourt (1995), sought to broaden the theoretical framework regarding the social determination and of the health-illness process. He defined the latter as that which, despite expressing itself concretely in individuals, also focuses on how human groups to which the individual belongs live, feed, educate, rest, recreate and organise themselves. The health-illness process refers to issues that are expressed in the singular dimension of being, which despite belonging to a community, has unique characteristics. Likewise, Lima (1994) points out that Laurell limits himself to analysing the forms of collective mani-festation of the disease, when it is necessary to acknowledge the form and specific way in which social processes and general determinations are expressed in the individual. It is also necessary, according to Lima, to know the relationship between the biological, including the psychological and the social. He argues that the studies carried out by Laurell are placed in the generality of the structural categories, where the individual occupies a reduced space. For the author, the genesis of diseases also involves individual dimensions, thus, necessary not only for explanation but also for prevention. In the case of capitalist societies, there is an open space, within certain structural limits, so individuals have different behaviours (Lima, 1994). Although these choices are clearly not free, they at least allow that concrete beha-viours differ, if not in quality in degree. Hence, different trajectories in life will show differ-ent forms of deterioration with a more or less broad margin that also depends of the individual strategies within structural constraints. The exclusive focus on collective forms of suffering eliminates the possibility of visualising how deterioration is established in the individual field. This leaves aside singular processes of health-illness, in addition to practical processes of resistance and transformation existing within society, which are built from individual strategies or small groups (Fernandes, 2003).

Barreto and Alves (1994) also discuss the tension between the collective and the indi-vidual in epidemiology. They acknowledge that the approach adopted by epidemiology to understand the collective presupposes its social determination. Even when historically inherited structural circumstances exist, the individuals monitor their actions in interactive processes, negotiating, adapting and modifying meanings and contexts. From this perspective, epidemiology denies essential aspects of the human collective: the universe of meanings, motives, aspirations, attitudes, values and believes (Barreto & Alves, 1994). These authors emphasise the need to overcome both perspectives through a synthesis that contemplates the objectivity of the structures, as well as the subjectivity of individual practices.

This article returns to the proposals that began to develop from 1990, with the designation of 'ethnoepidemiology' or 'sociocultural epidemiology', suggesting a superseding understanding of developments which, like the previous ones, focus on the social production of disease identifying the economic as the main determinant. These perspectives will try to address the multiple 'determinations' or constraints, both at the level of personal trajectories and structural conditions.

'Ethno' epidemiologies

Almeida Filho is one of the main precursor advocates of 'ethnoepidemiology', which he also refers to as the 'epidemiology of the way of life'. The author argues that it is not about creating explicative models and combining them with sociocultural variables. It is not a mere question of granting a certain place to the social, within models of illnesses epidemiologically conceived. Instead, it recognises the belonging of health-illness phenomena to the social processes as an ethno-epidemiological totality.

The prefix 'ethno' links this perspective to the microanalytic approach provided by ethnography, seeking to recognise the worldview of one who is defined as a 'cultural other'. On this, the proposal is close to the arguments raised by Mitchell G. Weiss from Basel University, Switzerland. 'Cultural epidemiology' emerged from this institute, and it is methodologically based on the emic interview, which refers to the local concepts of disease and implies collaboration between anthropology and epidemiology. Some key concepts of anthropology are used from this perspective, such as the emic/etic distinction. Linguist Kenneth Pike has done some of this work when differentiating phonemics–minimal units of meaning in a particular language, in that sense refers to local perspective–and phonetics, which refers to the acoustic reality, or external perspective. The differentiation between disease and illness is another key distinction that comes from medical anthropology. The first refers to sickness in biomedical terms, and the second to the meaning, experience, and behaviour of sickness from the emic perspective, which is used to examine patterns of distress, perceived causes, and help seeking (Weiss, 2001, p. 17). This perspective is framed in a culturalist anthropology, where the anthropologist acts as translator or intermediary between the categories and, local and professional concepts. In this sense, 'cultural epidemiology', as presented from this perspective, would seek to identify syndromes or health problems from the local perspective (of those who suffer it) making them possible to be approached from a medical or biomedical perspective. There is a risk of medicalizing suffering in this perspective. A clear example of this is formulated in Weiss' article (2001), when he argues that the research must be oriented towards investigating problems of mental health that might be incorporated to future editions of the Manual of Diagnostics and Treatments in Mental Health (DMH). This means a medicalisation and psychiatrization of mental suffering, from a perspective which excludes other health determinants like, for example, living conditions. Doing so risk the 'culturalizing' (or attributing to culture) of what in fact concerns, among other things, situations of economic inequality and of power or access to education or work. Considering the works conducted in Bangladesh, India, Malawi, Ghana, among others (see Swiss Tropical Institute, 2004), a question could be raised about whether disease is culturally constructed or if cultural reality is clinically constructed. That is, is it an inter-cultural dialogue or a manipulation of the local knowledge towards the biomedical perspective, where the latter is not problematised.

In contrast, Almeida Filho's proposal returns to concepts of epidemiology, from a critical perspective. When referring to 'risk factors' he points out that these do not exist beyond their statistical, epidemiologic and clinical significance. Furthermore, he argues that epidemiology should be open to the research of the symbolical aspects of risk determinants. Considering the complex, subjective and contextual nature of the relationship between health-disease and social process, the author suggests focussing less on the classic approach to 'risk factors' and more on 'fragilization models', which are more sensitive to symbolic specificities and the interactive character of the relationships between subjects and their cultural and sociohistorical environment. The symbolic would include the identification and description of discomfort, and the explanation regarding its origin and the actions oriented towards palliating or enduring that problem (which could be added to the approach of cultural epidemiology in the operationalisation that makes the concept of illness). However, this research will be broadened to include the relational, the environment and the particular sociohistorical contexts. Therefore, the intention is not to make a translation towards biomedicine, but understanding it in its own terms, seeking to identify actions that weaken health to attenuate deteriorating processes, as well as strengthening those actions that are protective. It must be considered that many answers that could be interpreted as 'cultural' must be understood as the result of historical processes and socio-environmental changes. Hence, they are cultural responses in conditions that people do not choose, such as a context of poverty, lack of access to education, work, drinking water, or an environment suitable for human life. From this perspective, one can argue that any event or social process, to represent a potential source of risk to health needs to be in resonance with an epidemiological structure of the human collectives. This relationship is not exclusively about the external action of an aggressive environmental element, as suggested in the metaphor of factors-producing-risks, nor the internalised reaction of a susceptible host. It is a system (totalised, interactive, procedural) of pathological effects (Almeida Filho, 1992a, 1992b, 2000). Therefore, it requires models capable of approaching the relationship among subjects and their bio-cultural and socio-historical environments.

If one takes this contextual approach to its logical conclusion, it is possible to argue that 'risk factors' are nothing more than an expression of the 'way of life' of the population groups under study. 'Way of life', which can be thought of as a wide and fundamental condition determinant of the health-disease relationship, is mediated by two dimensions: 'way of life' itself and living conditions (Possas, 1989). Hence, 'way of life' must be seen as a theoretical construct that does not merely include the individual components of health but also goes beyond to include sociohistorical dimensions, encompassing divisions of social class and culture, and taking consideration of the symbolic aspects of everyday life in society.

There is an opening for ethnographic research to address unexplored issues and model new scientific objects in the field of collective health. This could be achieved with the development of ethnoepidemiology. This discipline is not about the application of the epidemiological methodology to transcultural research in health, nor the introduction of ethno-models into the explanatory approach to risk. The ethnoepidemiological perspective starts primarily with self-reflection, acknowledging the sociohistorical character of the epidemiological discipline itself. It requires the construction of interpretative models of the health-disease process capable of integrating both perspectives through the application of methodological strategies that competently combine the quantitative and qualitative approaches into a single ethnoepidemiological strategy. One of its central assumptions is that health-disease phenomena are social processes and, conceived as such, they are historic, complex, fragmented, conflictive, dependent, ambiguous and uncertain. (Almeida Filho, 1992a, 2000). As Norma González González (2000) rightly points out, it is not simply about changing the statistical representation of the phenomenon. It must reach a conceptual development that allows understanding of the historical and social base of unequal distribution of health in human populations. It is a discipline whose ultimate purpose is to transform concrete realities of health.

Sociocultural epidemiology

Those who refer to sociocultural epidemiology highlight the necessary integration of the methods, techniques and theory of medical anthropology and epidemiology (Álvarez Hernández, 2008; Haro, 2010; Hersch-Martínez, 2013; Hersch-Martínez & Haro, 2007; Menéndez 1990, 2008, 2009). A core part of this proposal is centred in the recommendation of joining quantitative and qualitative methods, from the conformation of interdisciplinary teams to study the multiple forms (biological, behavioural, cultural, political) in which the process of health, disease and care express themselves, and not only the clinical or statistical manifestation of the illness. Thus, it seeks to recover the historical and sociocultural nature of health problems, researching how human groups are organised to address the health-disease process, particularly in those settings in which health inequality and vulnerability are more evident. The combination of quantitative and qualitative techniques supposes the methodological need of creating indicators with cultural, social and biological pertinence, but also with sufficient empirical validity. Hence, the data for their construction are not subject exclusively to the statistical value they possess, but also to the feasibility of their collection and the acceptance of the subjects (be they individuals or populations) with whom they work (Álvarez, 2008).

From the Latin American socio-epidemiological perspective, the subject will be considered not only as a unit of description and analysis or, as it has traditionally been considered: that is, the 'subject of study'. It will also be included as a *transforming agent*, which produces and reproduces social structure and meanings. In this approach, work is carried out using relational approaches, which seeks to recognise each of the significative actors in relation to a given problem and identify the form in which they relate to each other. Such links will allow the identification of the different factors that operate with respect to a given problem and incorporate the opinion of the conglomerate of significant social actors. Thus, to address health problems in communities implies a political and ideological commitment in which the effective participation of the population takes place. It is not only about regaining the other's rationality, but to include the needs, objectives and decisions of social actors themselves so they assume the projects regarding specific problems as their own (Menéndez, 2008).

Social epidemiology becomes an integrating operative and analytical referent, whose main objective is to apply different methods to approximate of the multifactorial and collective dimension of diseases, taking as one of its axes the category of 'avoidable damage'. This concept must be understood by identifying in the determinants of the disease the multiple factors that occur in the pathological expression, as well as the 'causes of the causes'. This involves the limitation of damage, but also reflects how popular perceptions about vulnerability relate with the production of knowledge regarding risk and the design of integral actions destined to its reduction. (Hersch-Martínez, 2013; Hersch-Martínez & Haro, 2007). Hence, one asks to what extent modern epidemiology identifies as risk factor is of social or cultural matrix to focus on the risk scenarios from where that and other factors emerge. The importance of sustaining as an instrumental purpose the understanding of how society responds to the health-disease process, and how this knowledge can serve to prevent, control or mitigate avoidable damages at the collective level must be highlighted (Álvarez, 2008).

From the framework of social epidemiology, one not only will investigate the explanatory models of diseases generated outside the biomedical paradigm, but also its epidemiological transcendence in terms of 'avoidable damage'. In this paradigm, prevention and care are prioritised, as well as essential social actors. Furthermore, one will contemplate not only the challenges involved in promoting health actions from specificities and local perspectives, but also what are the political obstacles inherent in those actions. Finally, it will not only formulate categories of impact measurement, but also consider the type and quality of social scenarios that arise from the impact (Hersch-Martínez, 2013).

Sociocultural epidemiology is thought of as a conceptual and applicative tool based on different descriptive and analytical strategies, which are selected based on the nature of the health problem being studies (Hersch-Martínez & Haro, 2007; Haro, 2010; Hersch-Martínez, 2013). Unlike Almeida Filho (1992b), who highlights the need for a new 'ethnoepidemiological' paradigm, Menéndez (2009) argues that it is not necessary to develop a new paradigm for the exercise of a social epidemiology. Sociocultural epidemiology does not seek, at least in principle, to develop a new scientific discipline. However, Hersch-Martínez (2013) recommends that the development and foundation of a new epidemiological theory and practice requires expanding and deepening its scope, without distancing itself from the contributions of biomedical research, integrating them with the results of the social sciences in the same field of knowledge to generate a synthesised view of health-related phenomena. In the methodological field, this implies significant changes in the formation of human resources, as well as a knowledge dialogue focused on the specific nature of the problems rather than disciplines.

Is a new episteme necessary?

By placing oneself in the field of Collective Health and returning to the criticisms of modern epidemiology–the main starting point–it is necessary to problematise the episteme in which the sciences are based, starting from a clear differentiation between nature/culture, and biological/social (Samaja, 2004). Biologization, individualisation, quantification and generalisation–the main criticisms of modern epidemiology–are only possible from such episteme. The alternative proposals immediately refer us to the consideration of non-Western epistemes, which decolonial theory labels as 'epistemes-other'. This perspective can be identified in Colombia, in relation to the so-called 'intercultural epidemiology', as a 'strategy that allows to know the epidemiological profile of the multiethnic and multicultural reality according to the different epistemes associated with health and disease processes'. Furthermore, this strategy allows the organisation of health services from an intercultural perspective (Portela, 2014, p. 249). Here, the recognition of diversity implies an equitable valuation of 'epistemes-other' or forms of knowing–comprehension, signification and action–of societies with dissimilar logics to which biomedical rationality underlies. Portela (2014) suggests, as a point of departure for the analysis, the global dimension of ethnicity, before the traditional divisions of anthropology (ie economy, social organisation, health, etc), since it could not speak of an indigenous medical system as such, but a culture of health. The latter is not limited to therapeutic, medical practices, classification systems, thoughts or philosophical conceptions, which can only be understood within a 'project of ethnicity'. To think a medical system as established by modernity, from this perspective, would be theoretically and methodologically inadequate. An intercultural epidemiology would be developed within the framework of a model of intercultural health services that address the ways of life of indigenous communities, to its peculiar ecological and environmental conditions, incorporating as theoretic-methodological research strategy the dialogue and negotiation of cultural meanings among health teams and communities around health and disease, life and death, healing and care. It requires some degree of conceptual and financial flexibility to be able to adapt the actions together with the authorities of those territories (Portela, 2008, 2014; Puerta, 2004).

From this perspective, as well as from ethno-epidemiology, the need arises to think from an 'episteme-other'. For that reason, one risks to think of epistemes, even ontologies that problematise the attribution of a 'natural' character, external, objective and independent of human action, to the biological or so-called 'natural'. Malnutrition is one such example: can it be treated as a merely physical problem? Considering the production and availability of food, is it environmental? Is malnutrition exclusively social or sociocultural? Or is it socioeconomic? Isolating malnutrition as a problem, or cutting it from one edge or another eliminates the possibility of seeing the problem with all its complexity. By denying a human character to nature, the episteme of science clearly separates the latter from culture, and it should not be forgotten that the episteme of science is the result of particular sociohistorical processes that enabled scientific development, which does not mean that it is scientific. Separating nature from culture is unthinkable, if one resorts to epistemes belonging to diverse indigenous populations from Latin America, which have favoured the development of other forms of knowledge. When referring to the worldview of Amazonian groups, Descola (1996) points out that such differentiation does not exist. Animals, plants, landscapes, stones, and even the stars receive human attributes and characteristics. They have a soul, and are conceived and treated as persons. In this sense, he is arguing that nature is a cultural construction. It filters, codifies and reorganises entities and primary properties from materials that culture has not provided itself. As the natural environment is anthropized and in varying degrees, its existence as an autonomous entity is a philosophical fiction (Descola, 1996, 2005, 2012).

Final comments

The matters addressed in this article show that there is still much debate in relation to the development of the socio/ethno-epidemiologies. The proposal in this paper identifies the need to think from a different episteme, which enables the consideration of overlapping and juxtaposed ecological factors as processes of socio-environmental change that, starting from the current situation, consider broader factors such as the trajectory and history of groups, and their way of life. The latter is considered as an instance that integrates living conditions and lifestyles as constitutive of the environment they occupy. Therefore, ethnographic research, focused on studying the occurrence of the disease in community context, with an analysis of the traditional knowledge and practices, as well as the way in which different factors of socio-environmental change affect it, should provide tools that contribute to an integral understanding of the problem from an episteme that does not limit the conceptions of health-disease in the medical sciences.

It is necessary to find a methodological approach where none of the aspects that make the health-disease-care process are overlooked, that allows an explanation of the 'real' processes in the community/social group/ethnicity, and that results in working with communities (which is not the same as imposing external categories on communities) (Sy, 2013).

In principle, this paper agrees with authors such as E. Menéndez, Armando Haro and Hersch Martínez regarding the need to start developing a sociocultural epidemiology, from the integration of theories, methods and techniques that come from epidemiology and medical anthropology. However, the goal must be the development of a paradigm that escapes the dichotomies reproduced by modernity by distinguishing between nature/culture, science/politics or ideology, among others. We work with 'objects-subjects' that manifest in ways that resist conventional structures. Hence, an approach is necessary to overcome impenetrable classifications, taxonomies and dichotomies. We must overcome the rigidity implied by the forms of describing, analysing and naming the epochal and disciplinary reality. What we suggest is to develop a matrix of knowledge that enables the creation of new 'objects' and more creative modalities of approaching problems. The field of collective health means occupying an interstitial space that seeks to overcome the dichotomous, taxonomic and classificatory thinking that distinguishes between scientific/non-scientific, individual/collective, health/disease, female/male, among others. We consider that a socio/ethno-epidemiology that lets us move between different cultures, ecologies, epistemes and ontologies as way of learning, dialoguing and accounting for events that affect health is paramount to secure a field like collective health. We must overcome the 'inter' and 'transdisciplinary' to give rise to a body of knowledge of its own, epistemically part of the limitations, criticisms and needs that emerge within the field itself and, consistent with its academic project, management and practices that respond to the demands and needs of local populations.

Notes

1. "La epidemiología enfrenta sus límites".
2. "Por uma epidemiologia da saúde coletiva"

3. *Salud Colectiva.*
4. "Por una epidemiología con más números".
5. "Epidemiología sin números".
6. "Por una epidemiología con (más que) números: cómo superar la falsa oposición cuantitativo cualitativo"

Acknowledgements

To the National Council of Scientific and Technical Investigations (CONICET). To the colleagues at the Institute of Collective Health because I learnt a lot from the discussions we shared, and to Eduardo Menéndez for his generous and committed teachings.

Disclosure statement

No potential conflict of interest was reported by the authors.

Funding

This work was supported by Consejo Nacional de Investigaciones Científicas y Técnicas.

References

Almeida Filho, N. (1992a). *Epidemiología sin números. Una introducción crítica a la ciencia epidemiológica.* Quito: Serie PALTEX. Organización Panamericana de la Salud, OPS/OMS.

Almeida Filho, N. (1992b). Por una etnoepidemiología. Esbozo de un nuevo paradigma epidemiológico. *Cuadernos Médico Sociales, 61*, 43–47.

Almeida Filho, N. (1993). La práctica teórica de la epidemiología social en América Latina. *Salud y Cambio, 10*(3), 25–31.

Almeida Filho, N. (2007). Por una epidemiología con (más que) números: cómo superar la falsa oposición cuantitativo cualitativo. [Editorial]. *Salud Colectiva, 3*(3), 229–233.

Almeida Filho, N., y Silva Paim, J. (1999). La crisis de la salud pública y el movimiento de la salud colectiva en Latinoamérica. *Cuadernos Médico Sociales, 75*, 5–30.

Almeida-Filho, N. (2000). *La ciencia tímida. Ensayos de deconstrucción de la Epidemiología.* Buenos Aires: Lugar Editorial.

Álvarez Hernández, G. (2008). Limitaciones metodológicas de la epidemiología moderna y una alternativa para superarlas: la epidemiología sociocultural. *Región y Sociedad, 20*(2), 51–75. Retrieved from http://www.redalyc.org/articulo.oa?id=10209803.

Barata, R. B., y Barreto, M. L. (1996). Algumas questões sobre o desenvolvimento da epidemiologia na América Latina. *Ciênc Saúde Coletiva, 1*, 70–79.

Barreto, M. I., & Alves, P. C. (1994). O coletivo versus o individual na epidemiologia: contradição o síntese? In: Qualidade de vida: compromisso histórico da epidemiologia. Belo Horizonte-Rio de Janeiro, p. 129–135.

Barreto, M. L. (1998). Por uma epidemiologia da saúde coletiva. *Revista Brasileira de Epidemiologia, 1*(2), 123–125. doi:10.1590/S1415-790X1998000200003

Betancourt, O. (1995). *Teoría y práctica de la salud de los trabajadores. La salud y el trabajo: Reflexiones teórico metodológicas.* Quito: Centro de Estudios y Asesoría en Salud, CEAS. Organización Panamericana de la Salud, OPS/OMS.

Bourdieu, P., Chamboredon, J. C., & Passeron, J. C. (2008). *El oficio de sociólogo.* Buenos Aires: Siglo XXI.

Breilh, J. (1995). Epidemiology's role in the creation of a humane world: Convergences and divergences among the schools. *Social Science & Medicine, 41*(7), 911–914. Retrieved from http://hdl.handle.net/10644/3286

Breilh, J. (1997). A epidemiologia na humanização da vida: convergências e desencontros das correntes. In R. B. Barata, M. L. Barreto, N. Almeida Filho, & R. P. Veras (Eds.), *Equidade e saúde: contribuições da epidemiologia* (pp. 23–37). Rio de Janeiro: FIOCRUZ/ABRASCO.

Breilh, J., & Granda, E. (1986). Los nuevos rumbos de la epidemiología. En: Duarte E. Ciencias sociales y salud en la América Latina. Tendencias y perspectivas. Organización Panamericana de la Salud (OPS). Organización Mundial de la Salud (OMS).

Descola, P. (1996). *Nature and society: Anthropological perspectives*. Londres: Routledge.

Descola, P. (2005). *Las lanzas del crepúsculo. Relatos jíbaros. Alta amazonia*. España: Fondo de Cultura Económica.

Descola, P. (2012). *Más allá de naturaleza y cultura*. Buenos Aires: Amorrortu.

Diez Roux, A. V. (2004). Genes, individuos, sociedad y epidemiología. In H. Spinelli (Comp.), *Salud Colectiva. Cultura, instituciones y subjetividad. Epidemiología, gestión y políticas* (pp. 71–81). Buenos Aires: Lugar Editorial.

Diez Roux, A. V. (2007). En defensa de una epidemiología con números. [Editorial]. *Salud Colectiva, 3*(2), 117–119.

Fernandes, R. C. P. (2003). Uma leitura sobre a perspectiva etnoepidemiológica. *Ciência & Saúde Coletiva, 8*(3), 765–774.

Frenk, J. (1992). La nueva Salud Pública. In *La crisis de la salud pública: reflexiones para el debate* (pp. 75–93). Washington, DC: Organización Panamericana de la Salud OPS – Publicación Científica. 540.

González González, N. (2000). Epidemiología y salud pública frente al proyecto neoliberal en México. *Papeles de Población, 25*, 207–225. Retrieved from http://www.redalyc.org/articulo.oa?id=11202510

Haro, J. A. (Ed.). (2010). *Epidemiología Sociocultural. Un diálogo en torno a su sentido, métodos y alcances*. Buenos Aires: Lugar Editorial.

Hersch-Martínez, P. (2013). Epidemiología sociocultural: una perspectiva necesaria. *Salud Publica de Mexico, 55*, 512–518. Retrieved from http://www.scielosp.org/pdf/spm/v55n5/v55n5a9.pdf

Hersch-Martínez, P., y Haro, J. A. (2007). *¿Epidemiología sociocultural o antropología médica? Algunos ejes para un debate disciplinar*. Tarragona: VII Coloquio REDAM. Retrieved from http://www.colson.edu.mx:8080/portales/portales218/epidemiologia%20sociocultural.pdf

Krieger, N. (1994). Epidemiology and the web of causation: Has anyone seen the spider? *Social Science & Medicine, 39*, 887–903. doi:10.1016/0277-9536(94)90202-X

Laurell, A. C. (1983). A saúde-doença como processo social. In E. D. Nunes (Org.), *Medicina Social: aspectos históricos e teóricos* (pp. 133–158). São Paulo: Global Ed.

Liborio, M. (2013). ¿Por qué hablar de Salud Colectiva? *Review(s) Méd Rosario, 79*, 136–141.

Lima, F. (1994). *Ergonomia e LER: como entender o processo de individuação da doença*. Belo Horizonte: Fundacentro (Mimeo).

Long, A. F. (1993). *Understanding health and disease: Towards a knowledge base for public health action*. Leeds: University of Leeds.

McMichael, A. J. (1995). The health of persons, populations and planets: Epidemiology comes full circle. *Epidemiology (Cambridge, Mass.), 6*(6), 633–636. Retrieved from http://journals.lww.com/epidem/Citation/1995/11000/The_Health_of_Persons,_Populations,_and_Planets_.13.aspx

McMichael, A. J. (1999). Prisoners of the proximate: Loosening the constraints on epidemiology in an age of change. *American Journal of Epidemiology, 149*(10), 887–897. Retrieved from http://aje.oxfordjournals.org/content/149/10/887.full.pdf+html

Menéndez, E. L. (1990). Antropología médica en México. Hacia la construcción de una epidemiología sociocultural. In *Antropología médica Orientaciones, desigualdades y transacciones* (pp. 24–49). México: CIESAS.

Menéndez, E. L. (2008). Epidemiología sociocultural: propuestas y posibilidades. *Región y Sociedad, 20*(2), 5–50. Retrieved from http://www.redalyc.org/articulo.oa?id=10209802

Menéndez, E. L. (2009). *De Sujetos, saberes y estructuras. Introducción al enfoque relacional en el estudio de la Salud Colectiva*. Buenos Aires: Lugar Editorial.

Paim, J. S. (1992). La salud colectiva y los desafíos de la práctica. In *La crisis de la salud pública: reflexiones para el debate* (pp. 151–167). Washington, DC: OPS. Publicación Científica 540.

Paim, J. S. (2011). *Desafíos para la Salud Colectiva en el siglo XXI*. Buenos Aires: Lugar Editorial.

Pearce, N. (1996). Traditional epidemiology, modern epidemiology, and public health. *American Journal of Public Health, 86*(5), 678–683. doi:10.2105/AJPH.86.5.678

Pearce, N. (2007). Commentary: The rise and rise of corporate epidemiology and the narrowing of epidemiology's vision. *International Journal of Epidemiology, 36*(4), 713–717. doi:10.1093/ije/dym152

Pearce, N. (2008). Corporate influences on epidemiology. *International Journal of Epidemiology, 37* (1), 46–53. doi:10.1093/ije/dym270

Portela, H. (2008). *La epidemiología intercultural. Argumentaciones, requerimientos y propuestas*. Popayán: Editorial Universidad del Cauca.

Portela, H. (2014). Epistemes – otras: contribución potencial a la organización intercultural de la salud en Colombia. *Review(s) University Salud, 16*(2), 246–263.

Possas, C. (1989). *Epidemiologia e Sociedade*. São Paulo: Hucitec.

Puerta, C. (2004). Roles y estrategias de los gobiernos indígenas en el sistema de salud colombiano. *Revista Colombiana de Antropología, 40*, 85–121.

Rothman, K. J. (2007). The rise and fall of epidemiology, 1950–2000 A.D. *International Journal of Epidemiology, 36*(4), 708–710. doi:10.1093/ije/dym150

Samaja, J. (2004). *Epistemología de la Salud. Reproducción social, subjetividad y transdisciplina*. Buenos Aires: Lugar Editorial.

Shy, C. M. (1997). The failure of academic epidemiology: Witness for the prosecution. *American Journal of Epidemiology, 145*(6), 479–487. Retrieved from http://aje.oxfordjournals.org/content/145/6/479.full.pdf+html

Silva Ayçaguer, L. C. (1997). Hacia una cultura epidemiológica revitalizada.*Dimension Human, 1* (5), 23–33.

Silva Ayçaguer, L. C. (2005). Una ceremonia estadística para identificar factores de riesgo. *Salud Colectiva, 1*(3), 309–322. Retrieved from https://www.researchgate.net/publication/237479082_HACIA_UNA_CULTURA_EPIDEMIOLOGICA_REVITALIZADA. doi:10.18294/sc.2005.49

Sousa Campos, G. (2000). Saúde pública e saúde coletiva: campo e núcleo de saberes e práticas. *Ciência y Saúde Coletiva, 5*(2), 219–230. doi:10.1590/S1413-81232000000200002

Sterne, J. A. C., & Smith, G. D. (2001). Sifting the evidence—what's wrong with significance tests? *BMJ: British Medical Journal, 322*(7280), 226–231.

Susser, M., & Susser, E. (1996a). Chosing a future for epidemiology. Part I: Eras and paradigms. *American Journal of Public Health, 86*(5), 668–673. doi:10.2105/AJPH.86.5.668

Susser, M., & Susser, E. (1996b). Choosing a future for epidemiology: II. From black box to Chinese boxes and ecoepidemiology. *American Journal of Public Health, 86*(5), 674–677. doi:10.2105/AJPH.86.5.674

Swiss Tropical Institute. (2004). Section 8. Cultural epidemiology. *Swiss Tropical Institute Report* 2003–2004. Retrieved from http://www.swisstph.ch/fileadmin/user_upload/Pdfs/Annual_Reports_STI/BR2003-2004/rreport8.pdf

Sy, A. (2009). Una revisión de los estudios en torno a enfermedades gastrointestinales. En busca de nuevas alternativas para el análisis de los procesos de salud- enfermedad". *Salud Colectiva, 5*(1), 65–78. doi:10.18294/sc.2009.230

Sy, A. (2013). Who defines culturally acceptable health access? Universal rights, healthcare politics and the problems of two Mbya-Guarani communities in the Misiones province, Argentina. *Health, Culture and Society, 4*(1), 1–19. doi:10.5195/hcs.2013.24

Taubes, G., y Mann, C. C. (1995). Epidemiology faces its limits. *Science, 269*, 164–169. doi:10.1126/science.7618077

Testa, M. (1992). Salud pública: acerca de un sentido y significado. In *La crisis de la salud pública: reflexiones para el debate* (pp. 205–229). Washington, DC: OPS. Publicación Científica 540.

Testa, M., & Paim, J. S. (2010). Memoria e Historia: diálogo entre Mario Testa y Jairnilson Silva Paim. *Salud Colectiva, 6*(2), 211–227. Retrieved from http://revistas.unla.edu.ar/saludcolectiva/article/view/367/387

Weiss, M. G. (2001). Cultural epidemiology: An introduction and overview. *Anthropology & Medicine*, *8*(1), 5–29. Retrieved from http://www.who.int/social_determinants/strategy/ QandAs/es/. doi:10.1080/13648470120070980

World Health Organization. (2005). Comisión sobre Determinantes Sociales en Salud. Retrieved from http://www.who.int/social_determinants/strategy/QandAs/es/.

Mitigating social and health inequities: Community participation and Chagas disease in rural Argentina

Ignacio Llovet, Graciela Dinardi and Fernando G. De Maio

Chagas disease (CD) causes 12,500 deaths annually in Latin America. As a neglected disease primarily associated with poverty, it is a major driver of health inequity. Argentina's efforts to control vector transmission have been unsuccessful. Using new survey data ($n = 400$ households), we compare the social patterning of the burden of CD by examining socio-demographic predictors of self-reported CD and the presence of *vinchucas* in two areas of rural northern Argentina known to have experienced different interventions in surveillance and control. Our analyses suggest that Avellaneda, an area known for horizontal intervention strategies which nurture community participation is quite distinct from Silípica, an area which has experienced a vertical intervention strategy since 1990. Avellaneda has higher level of self-reported Chagas infection and lower level of *vinchuca* presence; Silípica has pronounced and statistically significant differences patterned by the head of household's level of educational attainment. A greater awareness of the disease and its transmission, along with community mobilisation and spraying, may bring about more self-reported CD and less *vinchuca* presence in Avellaneda than in Silípica. This suggests that strategies based on community participation may be effective in reducing the social patterning of the burden of disease, even in poor places.

Introduction

Neglected infectious diseases (NIDs) are a heterogeneous group of parasitic and bacterial diseases whose persistence is closely associated with environmental and social conditions (Holveck et al. 2007, Mathers et al. 2007, Hotez et al. 2008). NIDs are primarily diseases of poverty (Ault 2007, Crompton and Pearson 2008), affecting marginalised segments of populations with limited access to water, housing and education (Hunt 2007). They are also diseases that impose significant social and financial burdens on individuals, families and communities (Hotez et al. 2007). As a result, NIDs are best understood as both outcomes and key drivers of the profound inequities that exist in Latin America.

Chagas disease (CD) ranks among the most significant NIDs in Latin America (Hotez et al. 2007). Recent World Health Organisation (WHO) estimates suggest that more than 7 million people are infected with CD in the region, with most infected people living in settings of economic marginalisation (TDR/SWG 2009). CD is largely asymptomatic and under-diagnosed (Lugones 2001). It is estimated to produce 12,500 annual deaths in Latin America (OPS/WHO/NTD/IDM 2006). It is also a significant cause of morbidity (WHO 2002), work disability and increased health-care costs (Dias 2007). A potential clinical consequence of *Trypanosoma cruzi* (*T. cruzi*) is chagasic cardiomyopathy which may lead to heart failure and sudden death (WHO 2002).

Chagas disease (CD) in Argentina

There are three routes of disease transmission: vectorial, congenital and through blood transfusion, with vectorial transmission being the most frequent (Prata 2001). This is clearly the case in Argentina, where CD is primarily caused by the protozoan *T. cruzi*, borne by a triatomine bug commonly referred to as *vinchuca*. *Vinchucas* colonise sub-standard dwellings (WHO 2002, Dias 2007) and also pose significant concerns in rural areas characterised by close contact between humans and animals. It is through this colonisation that 'man becomes an active component of the epidemiological chain of CD' (TDR/SWG 2009, p. 9, our translation). The conditions that make this colonisation possible are economic under-development, inadequate housing and the inequitable distribution of resources (Briceño-León 1990, Bastien 1998).

Spraying of insecticides and entomological surveillance have been the main epidemiological tools to control vectorial transmission (Segura 2002). During the 1960s and 1970s, national programmes for vector control were designed and launched (Dias et al. 2002). Since their inception, vector-control activities were attached to centralised and vertical structures conducted with a top–bottom approach. Occasionally, horizontal strategies involving primary health-care services (PHCS) in vectorial control were promoted; these often opened important opportunities for community participation as well (Segura 2002). Vector-control efforts proved successful as incidence of new infections by *T. cruzi* diminished by 70% between 1983 and 2000 (Moncayo 2003). However, this progress has been uneven. Brazil, Chile and Uruguay succeeded in interrupting vectorial disease transmission (TDR/SWG 2009), but Argentina failed in achieving that goal. Although Argentina carried out massive sprayings between 1960 and 1990 with a drastic reduction of *T. cruzi* prevalence, it never succeeded in its efforts to build an epidemiological surveillance system for the prevention and control of CD (Zaidemberg et al. 2004).

Since 1982, Argentina experienced important shifts between models and organisational strategies for dealing with CD. In a decentralisation process characterised by complex relationships between national and provincial programmes, these changes limited the country's ability to develop entomological and epidemio-logical surveillance in provinces particularly affected by *vinchucas* (Llovet and Dinardi 2006). This is the case in the province of Santiago del Estero, a highly endemic area. Starting in the early 1990s, National and Provincial Chagas Programmes (PCP) agreed to split the provincial territory to undertake control and prevention activities. The National Chagas Programme (NCP) was in charge of

24 out of 27 *departamentos* (a sub-provincial administrative unit, in Spanish), one of them Avellaneda (28°35′53.86″S, 62°56′47.11″W). Meanwhile, the PCP was left in charge of the remaining three, one of them Silípica (28°03′3.64″S, 64°13′30.86″W). As a consequence of this division of responsibilities, and because the PCP never committed to community participation as a tool for control and surveillance actions, a top–bottom approach prevailed in Silípica.

Community participation initiatives and primary health-care involvement have been developed in Argentina, but never in a systematic fashion. A consequence is that what may be called 'natural experiments' can be found in the country. This study compares the social patterning of the burden of CD by examining socio-demographic predictors of self-reported CD and the presence of *vinchucas* in two areas known to have experienced different strategies in surveillance and control.

Community participation in surveillance and disease control

Since the late nineteenth century, community participation in public health programmes has been shown to be successful in reducing the burden of infectious diseases, particularly in the context of weak states (Vaughan 1991, Manderson 1996). The aim of these experiences had been to encourage the population to adopt preventive measures in the absence of public health agencies. In a related but different vein, community participation in health, as a principle introduced by Declaration of Alma Ata is still a powerful concept in the international arena, where populations are expected to 'identify their own health priorities and implement appropriate strategies on that basis' (Espino et al. 2004, p. 4). This complex concept 'encompasses a spectrum of approaches and strategies' (Espino et al. 2004, p. 9), which can be summarised in the utilitarian and the empowerment perspectives (Morgan 2001).

The utilitarian approach sees community participation as a mean for goal achievement, allowing for effective and efficient programme implementation (Uphoff et al. 1998, Morgan 2001). In contrast, the empowerment approach considers community participation as an end in itself (Morgan 2001, Espino et al. 2004).

The utilitarian approach has been widely used in prevention and control programmes for some tropical and vector-borne diseases, including CD (Bryan et al. 1994, Briceño-León 2001, Espino et al. 2004). In the context of CD prevention and control, more active or more passive utilitarian approaches have been applied (Bryan et al. 1994). Reported benefits arising from community participation include vector-density reduction, increased cost-effectiveness of interventions and, in some cases, shrinking figures of *T. cruzi* transmission to humans (Bryan et al. 1994).

Pioneering community participation initiatives in 1985 was the María Project in Río Hondo, Santiago del Estero, initiated by the National Ministry of Health. It was a horizontal intervention as PHCS were significantly involved in entomological surveillance (Chuit et al. 1992, Segura 2002). Furthermore, María Project surveyed knowledge on disease transmission and control methods, attitudes and inclinations of rural inhabitants regarding participation (Mercer 1988). Nonetheless, community participation was kept at a low level, as dwellers' main role was to grant access to their houses to be sprayed and to provide parental authorisation for serological studies of newborn babies. Thus, community participation was mostly passive (Bryan et al. 1994).

Between 1992 and 1998, Argentina launched a large national initiative to establish a vector surveillance system based on community participation, training community leaders and members for *Triatoma infestans* detection and house spraying (Chuit et al. 1992, Segura et al. 1994, Segura 2002). Within this framework, 77 participatory workshops were held in Avellaneda, organised by the NCP with local support. Following this development, in 2002 and 2003 social networks in Avellaneda with more than 300 participants were set up to support interventions and sprayings (Segura 2005). Community involvement was, in this case, mostly active (Bryan et al. 1994).

Thus, Avellaneda's history of control intervention differs from that experienced by other areas, including our second field site, Silípica. These differences reflected the approach undertaken by the NCP and the PCP. In Avellaneda, a horizontal intervention strategy with community participation had been applied by the NCP. In Silípica, a vertical intervention strategy was carried out by the PCP since 1990. In Avellaneda during 2003 and 2004, the NCP sprayed dwellings with the involvement of social networks and designed a framework for a bottom-up notification path. Serological surveillance was also carried out among the population that was under 14 years old. Thus, interventions with horizontal arrangements stretched out on and off in Avellaneda for a period of 10 years. After 2004, however, due to political instability, community participation was brought to a standstill.

Unlike Avellaneda, the scattered CD interventions in Silípica have to be traced far back in time. Between 1983 and 1985, serosurveys were conducted under PCP guidance. In 1994, PCP sprayed dwellings and no further control actions took place until 2006.

In light of the broad consensus among researchers and policy-makers that CD is intimately related to social conditions (WHO 2002, Dias 2007), we may expect that the process of community participation that characterises Avellaneda may yield benefits that may now be detected. Thus, a relevant research question is if community participation in a concrete experience of vector control and surveillance has been able to mitigate inequity in CD distribution in the population.

Methods

The two research sites are in Santiago del Estero, a CD endemic area. This is a poverty-stricken province where the most vulnerable sector are rural dispersed households experiencing a high level of unsatisfied basic needs (48%), higher than the overall rate for Argentina (31%; INDEC 2001).

Educational achievement in the province is low; 25% of the population older than 15 years has less than elementary-level education, almost doubling the figure at the national level (INDEC 2001). Also, 63% of population has no health insurance, relying only on a feeble public health-care system, surpassing the national figure, 48% (INDEC 2001). Between 2001 and 2005, 51 out of 76 acute cases of CD reported in Argentina were identified in Santiago del Estero (Ministerio de Salud 2002, 2005, 2006). Samples of rural households were drawn from two *departamentos*, Avellaneda and Silípica. Despite modest improvements (Gómez 2004), both Avellaneda and Silípica rank among the poorest *departamentos* in the country. The selection criterion sought to control for socio-demographic traits and economic similarity on the one hand and different interventions for CD control and surveillance that health authorities carried out during the last 15 years, on the other.

Data collection

A cross-sectional survey was carried out. Data gathering was done through a 63 closed- and open-ended questionnaire (available upon request). The survey's goal was to collect the following information: (1) socio-demographics (age, sex, relation to household head, education and occupation); (2) community participation in vectorial-transmission prevention and control (involvement in control and surveillance activities, *vinchuca* presence in the dwelling, attitude towards *vinchucas* when found, information sharing regarding vector detection, frequency of meetings with neighbours to discuss community matters and participation in community institutions); (3) health and health-care access (CD condition, serotests for pregnant women and children); and (3) domestic and household habits (years of dwelling occupancy, dwelling improvements, shuffling of furniture and household stuff, and beliefs related to their dwelling's infestation with *T. infestans*).

Sampling

A random sample of 400 rural households was drawn (Avellaneda, $N = 200$; Silípica, $N = 200$). Sample selection of households was done in two stages: selection of census segments and selection of households within each segment. A team of local interviewers and a field supervisor was trained using role-playing techniques to build rapport and rehearsing real-life situations by research-team members. Fieldwork took place between August and September 2006, i.e., 3 years after the community participation experience ended, and was greatly facilitated by the good response of key local people who acted as gatekeepers. Overall, the refusal rate was a satisfactory 7%. An informed consent letter was given to sampled householders or read aloud in case of illiteracy. This letter explained the reason for the study, and provided information on CD in the province. An institutional ethical committee reviewed and approved the research design. Data were processed and analysed using SPSS 17.0.

Data analysis

These analyses examine socio-demographic predictors of: (1) a household member having CD, and (2) the presence of *vinchucas* in the household. A two-step modelling process was used: first, bivariate models examine the relationship between each predictor and the dependent variable. This was followed by models that included all of the predictors, regardless of their significance in the bivariate stage. To enable a comparison of how predictors operated across the two localities, separate models were run for Avellaneda and Silípica. Results from the logistic regression models are presented through odds ratios (OR) and 95% confidence intervals (95% CI).

Results

Comparison of the two localities indicates important differences, with Avellaneda displaying a worse profile on key indicators (Table 1). Most notably, respondents from Avellaneda are more likely to indicate that a household member has CD (37.4% vs. 13.7% in Silípica, $\chi^2 = 26.06$, $p < 0.001$). Data from Avellaneda also indicate a higher proportion of households where the head of the household had little or no formal schooling (70.8% vs. 48.2% in Silípica, $\chi^2 = 20.53$, $p < 0.001$), and a somewhat greater reliance on the agricultural sector for employment. However, the presence of *vinchucas* was reported to be higher in Silípica.

The two areas differ with respect to households' participation in community activities (Table 2). Households in Avellaneda are more likely than households in Silípica to belong to a community network (20.6% vs. 5.5%, $\chi^2 = 19.91$, $p < 0.01$) and are far more likely to report meeting with neighbours to discuss problems (31.5% vs. 6.5%, $\chi^2 = 40.61$, $p < 0.01$). When asked what type of problems they discussed with neighbours, water issues/drought was the most common response in both localities.

Table 1. Description of the sample.

	Avellaneda		Silípica		Total		
	N	%	N	%	N	%	Significance
Dependent variables							
Household member with Chagas disease							
Yes	67	37.4	24	13.7	91	25.7	<0.001
No	112	62.6	151	86.3	263	74.3	
Presence of *vinchucas* in the household							
Yes	100	50.0	148	74.0	248	62.0	<0.001
No	100	50.0	52	26.0	152	38.0	
Independent variables							
Education							
Less than primary	138	70.8	93	48.2	231	59.5	<0.001
Primary or more	57	29.2	100	51.8	157	40.5	
Age (head of household, years)							
20–39	48	24.2	58	29.0	106	26.6	0.676
40–49	42	21.2	37	18.5	79	19.8	
50–64	54	27.3	56	28.0	110	27.6	
65 or more	54	27.3	49	24.5	103	25.9	
Sex (head of household)							
Female	33	16.7	43	21.5	76	19.1	0.220
Male	165	83.3	157	78.5	322	80.9	
Single-parent household?							
Yes	37	18.5	34	17.0	71	17.8	0.695
No	163	81.5	166	83.0	329	82.3	
Occupation (head of household)							
Agricultural sector	112	56.0	89	44.5	201	50.3	<0.05
Non-agricultural sectors	88	44.0	111	55.5	199	49.8	
Household size							
3 or less	61	30.5	45	22.5	106	26.5	<0.001
4 or 5	39	19.5	64	32.0	103	25.8	
6 or 7	57	28.5	42	21.0	99	24.8	
8 or more	43	21.5	49	24.5	92	23.0	

Note: Percentages may not add to 100% due to rounding. Significance values based on chi-square tests.

Table 2.   Participation in community activities, Avellaneda and Silípica.

	Avellaneda		Silípica		Total		
	N	%	*N*	%	*N*	%	Significance
Do you or does a member of your household…							
Actively participate in C & S workshops?							
Yes	26	13.0	0	0	26	6.5	<0.001
No	174	87.0	200	100	374	93.5	
Carry out activities to control *vinchucas* in your home?							
Yes	63	31.5	48	24.0	111	27.7	0.094
No	137	68.5	152	76.0	289	72.5	
If yes, are these activities supervised?							
Yes	13	20.6	0	0	13	11.7	<0.001
No	50	79.4	48	100	98	88.3	
Give notice when *vinchuca* is found?							
Yes	23	11.5	3	1.5	26	6.5	<0.001
No	177	88.5	197	98.5	374	93.5	
Attend meetings at the local school?[a]							
Yes	103	60.9	125	68.7	228	65.0	0.129
No	66	39.1	57	31.3	123	35.0	
Participate in a community network?							
Yes	41	20.6	11	5.5	52	13.1	<0.001
No	158	79.4	188	94.5	346	86.9	
Attend meetings at church?							
Yes	98	49.2	111	55.8	209	52.5	0.192
No	101	50.8	88	44.2	189	47.5	
Attend meetings at the club?							
Yes	65	32.7	61	33.3	126	33.0	0.889
No	134	67.3	122	66.7	256	67.0	
Participate in activities at the hospital or health centre?							
Yes	20	10.1	13	6.6	33	8.4	0.220
No	179	89.9	183	93.4	362	91.6	
Meet with neighbours to discuss problems?							
Yes	63	31.5	13	6.5	76	19.0	<0.001
No	137	68.5	187	93.5	324	81.0	

[a]Asked only of households with children of school age.
Note: Percentages may not add to 100% due to rounding. Significance values based on chi-square tests.

CD prevention and spraying were reported by a few households in Avellaneda and none in Silípica as the topic of discussion with neighbours. Importantly, only respondents from Avellaneda ($n = 26$) had participated in community workshops devoted to the surveillance and control of *vinchucas* (C & S workshops). Households in Avellaneda may also be more likely than households in Silípica to carry out activities to control *vinchucas* in their home (31.5% vs. 24.0%), although that difference was not statistically significant at the $p < 0.05$ level. Only households from Avellaneda reported receiving any kind of supervision of their *vinchuca* control activities. Similarly, almost all the households that report *vinchucas* to local authorities when found are from Avellaneda. Household participation in churches', clubs' and schools' activities was similar across both localities.

Table 3 presents the results of a series of regression models that examine the predictive power of demographic variables and household characteristics on the probability that a household reports a member with CD. Education is a statistically significant predictor in Silípica, with households where the head has little or no formal schooling having an increased probability of having a member with CD (OR = 4.03, 95% CI = 1.37–11.82). Women as the head of the household also displays predictive power of having a member with CD in Silípica (OR = 5.60, 95% CI = 1.10–28.57), but not in Avellaneda. Age of the head of the household does not display explanatory power in any of the models, nor does their occupation or single-parent status. Household size is also not a significant predictor, with the exception of very large households (eight or more members) in Avellaneda having an increased likelihood of having a member with CD.

Educational attainment of the head of the household displays a similar relationship when the presence of *vinchucas* is considered as the dependent variable (see Table 4); very little difference is observed within Avellaneda (OR = 1.09, 95% CI = 0.57–2.11), although it approaches significance in the Silípica models

Table 3. Logistic regression (predictors of having a household member with CD).

	Avellaneda				Silípica			
	Model 1: unadjusted		Model 2: adjusted		Model 3: unadjusted		Model 4: adjusted	
	OR	95% CI	OR	95% CI	OR	95% CI	OR	95% CI
Socio-demographics								
Education								
Primary or more	1.00	–	1.00	–	1.00	–	1.00	–
Less than primary	1.63	0.82–3.24	1.97	0.94–4.15	2.75	1.06–7.13	4.03	1.37–11.82
Age (head of household, years)								
20–39	1.00	–	1.00	–	1.00	–	1.00	–
40–49	1.13	0.46–2.73	0.88	0.33–2.34	0.71	0.20–2.54	0.43	0.10–1.84
50–64	0.99	0.42–2.33	1.05	0.42–2.66	0.71	0.23–2.18	0.43	0.11–1.66
65 or more	0.53	0.22–1.31	0.87	0.29–2.59	0.69	0.21–2.26	0.31	0.06–1.54
Sex (head of household)								
Male	1.00	–	1.00	–	1.00	–	1.00	–
Female	0.47	0.19–1.16	0.50	0.14–1.80	2.20	0.86–5.64	5.60	1.10–28.57
Single-parent household?								
No	1.00	–	1.00	–	1.00	–	1.00	–
Yes	0.54	0.24–1.24	0.66	0.26–1.69	1.86	0.67–5.17	0.43	0.09–2.17
Occupation (head of household)								
Non-agricultural sectors	1.00	–	1.00	–	1.00	–	1.00	–
Agricultural sector	1.17	0.63–2.15	0.93	0.46–1.91	0.81	0.34–1.93	0.96	0.28–3.26
Household size								
3 or less	1.00	–	1.00	–	1.00	–	1.00	–
4 or 5	1.89	0.74–4.85	1.42	0.48–4.22	1.44	0.34–6.14	1.43	0.28–7.24
6 or 7	2.24	0.98–5.15	1.52	0.54–4.29	2.80	0.67–11.78	2.49	0.44–14.16
8 or more	4.09	1.68–9.96	3.14	1.02–9.71	2.74	0.67–11.19	2.17	0.44–10.67

(OR $= 2.05$, 95% CI $= 0.99$–4.24). No other independent variable attains statistical significance in these models.

Discussion

Cross-sectional self-reported data on CD in the households and *vinchuca* presence reflect the history of epidemiological intervention in Avellaneda and Silípica. Our analyses suggest that Avellaneda, an area known for horizontal intervention strategies that nurtured community participation, is quite distinct from Silípica, an area that has experienced a vertical intervention strategy since 1990. Institutional arrangements involving national and sub-national levels of CD agencies played a key role in defining the intervention strategies that would be followed in Avellaneda and Silípica. Our data show that Avellaneda has a higher level of *known* CD, a lower level of *vinchuca* presence, whereas Silípica has pronounced and statistically significant differences patterned by the head of household's level of educational attainment. A greater awareness of the disease and its transmission, community mobilisation and

Table 4. Logistic regression (predictors of having *vinchucas* in the household).

	Avellaneda				Silípica			
	Model 1: unadjusted		Model 2: adjusted		Model 3: unadjusted		Model 4: adjusted	
	OR	95% CI	OR	95% CI	OR	95% CI	OR	95% CI
Socio-demographics								
Education								
Primary or more	1.00	–	1.00	–	1.00	–	1.00	–
Less than primary	0.99	0.54–1.84	1.09	0.57–2.11	1.75	0.91–3.38	2.05	0.99–4.24
Age (head of household, years)								
20–39	1.00	–	1.00	–	1.00	–	1.00	–
40–49	0.71	0.31–1.62	0.69	0.28–1.66	0.95	0.35–2.59	0.79	0.27–2.31
50–64	0.67	0.31–1.47	0.62	0.27–1.14	0.60	0.26–1.41	0.48	0.19–1.22
65 or more	0.78	0.36–1.70	0.71	0.28–1.83	0.59	0.25–1.42	0.38	0.13–1.11
Sex (head of household)								
Male	1.00	–	1.00	–	1.00	–	1.00	–
Female	0.51	0.24–1.11	0.42	0.15–1.17	1.43	0.63–3.22	2.00	0.63–6.41
Single-parent household?								
No	1.00	–	1.00	–	1.00	–	1.00	–
Yes	0.41	0.19–0.87	0.95	0.41–2.19	1.43	0.58–3.53	1.14	0.43–3.03
Occupation (head of household)								
Non-agricultural sectors	1.00	–	1.00	–	1.00	–	1.00	–
Agricultural sector	1.18	0.67–2.06	0.87	0.45–1.67	1.26	0.66–2.38	1.43	0.64–3.17
Household size								
3 or less	1.00	–	1.00	–	1.00	–	1.00	–
4 or 5	0.75	0.34–1.69	0.59	0.23–1.53	1.33	0.56–3.16	0.96	0.35–2.66
6 or 7	0.62	0.30–1.28	0.44	0.17–1.13	1.02	0.40–2.57	0.65	0.20–2.12
8 or more	0.83	0.38–1.82	0.63	0.27–1.73	1.25	0.50–3.13	0.95	0.31–2.85

spraying may bring about more self-reported CD and less *vinchuca* presence in Avellaneda than in Silípica.

Across our regression models, education displays an effect consistent with the literature on social determinants of health (CSDH 2008, Harling et al. 2008, De Maio et al. 2009), but it only attains statistical significance in the Silípica models predicting the presence of a household member reporting CD. These results may be a sign that Avellaneda's horizontal intervention strategy alleviates an important aspect of inequity (as marked by educational attainment of the head of the household). At the same time, our findings are consistent with existing work that emphasises the major impact that gender inequality has on the distribution of NIDs (Danis-Lozano et al. 2002, Manderson et al. 2009). Results from Silípica and Avellaneda indicate that horizontal prevention strategies may be associated with a decreased gender differential in CD. This suggests that horizontal intervention strategies based on rural community participation may be effective in reducing the social patterning of the burden of disease, even in poor places.

Our models suggest that educational differences are significant in Silípica but not Avellaneda for presence of a household reporting a member with CD. Additionally, female head of household is a significant predictor of CD in Silípica, but not Avellaneda. These patterns are repeated in the models predicting the presence of *vinchucas*, but without statistical significance for either education or sex of the head of the household. This weaker significance may be a reflection of the way in which the two dependent variables – household member with CD and *vinchuca* presence – interact with different levels of social organisation. On one hand, the self-reported presence of a member with CD may be more directly related to health care and prevention measures at the level of each individual household. On the other hand, self-reported *vinchuca* presence is susceptible to household-specific behaviour as well as environmental factors and collective action.

Fragility is a well-known feature of community participation experiences. That is less so, when it is led – initiated and developed – by external agents mainly in the case of vector-borne diseases (Espino et al. 2004). However, despite the advantage gained by an external orientation, this does not in itself guarantee that the participative experience will endure. Avellaneda's experience shows that sustainability of these endeavours is an issue. Factors such as low social capital of neglected populations (Dias 2001) and resistance by sub-national decision makers (Kahssay and Oakley 1999) collude in eroding community participation. This is particularly the case in Argentina, where implementation of community participation – with diverse degrees of intensity – has in some ways been a response to public health failures (Morel 2006) rather than a long-term structural strategy. After 2004, community actions in Avellaneda were brought to an end and a return to a vertical strategy was proposed, but this has not been immediately applied. Paradoxically, in Argentina, community participation terminology is widely used in public documents and as a keyword in the technical guidelines of the national health system (Llovet and Dinardi 2008). However, the potentiality of a co-operative interaction between horizontal and vertical arrangements has been poorly explored and applied.

There are several limitations to these analyses. Most notably, these include our use of self-reported measures and our reliance on cross-sectional, rather than longitudinal data. Available studies assume self-report as a *proxy* of health condition and can be found in the literature for different settings and diseases providing empirical support when measuring health and morbidities (Keating et al. 2005, Subramanian et al. 2009). However, no studies of self-report of CD have been found. This void may be attributed to its asymptomatic and under-diagnosed characteristics. Our own use of CD self-report departs from the former as we intend to capture the comparative distribution of disease awareness and information across households.

Regarding self-report of vector presence, self-report measures were previously used in rural Morelos, México, when potential risk factors for *Triatoma pallidipennis* domiciliary infestation were examined by Cohen et al. (2006). More importantly, a study conducted in Cuernavaca, Mexico, using combined methods ranging from specialised entomological observation to householder's reporting the presence of bugs inside or outside houses, concluded that householders were reliable informants, with 85% correlation between reported bug sightings and detection of infestation (Ramsey et al. 2005).

Self-reported health data should be subject to cautious treatment as dissonant relationships between these and other health indicators may occur (De Maio 2007). There may also exist clearly an element of reporting error, with tendencies that may lead to under-reporting (e.g., lack of knowledge, fear of stigma, social desirability) and over-reporting (e.g., acquiescence, or a respondent's tendency to answer questions in a way that they believe will be helpful to the interviewer). These limitations notwithstanding, we have no reason to believe that the patterning of responses would differ between areas in the same province; that is, under- and over-reporting should not be expected to be more pronounced in Silípica than in Avellaneda. Relative comparison of self-reported CD condition and *vinchuca* presence across the *departamentos* under study therefore may yield important insight.

Disaggregated longitudinal rather than cross-sectional data on socio-economic variables, like housing quality improvement, or knowledge and practices variables would also have enriched the analysis.

Conclusion

NIDs mainly affect poor rural populations, imposing social and financial burdens on individuals, families and communities. Not only does socio-economic inequality bring about health inequity but it is also reinforced by these health outcomes. In this way, NIDs such as CD are both outcomes and key drivers of the profound inequities that exist in countries like Argentina.

As a consequence of organisational arrangements reached by NCP and PCP, a definite horizontal strategy with community participation was applied in Avellaneda. This strategy played a role to lessen inequities in health outcomes. Our results indicate that in the case of CD, inequity amelioration can be experienced by vulnerable populations through community participation in surveillance activities. Some of the differences regarding households' involvement in health-related issues, e.g., prevention, may be attributed to horizontal participation *vis-à-vis* vertical intervention. This suggests that horizontal intervention strategies based on community participation may be effective in reducing the social patterning of the burden of disease, even in poor places. Nonetheless, excessive confidence on community-based horizontal models may lead to incomplete and frustrating experiences, particularly if it 'unloads' responsibility for health services from the state to marginalised populations. Future studies should explore how horizontal and vertical approaches may be integrated to best meet the population health challenges generated by neglected diseases such as CD.

Acknowledgements

The investigators wish to acknowledge the UNICEF/UNDP/World Bank/WHO–TDR for funding this research, to Dr Elsa Segura, to the communities of Avellaneda and Silípica and to faculties and students of Universidad Nacional de Santiago del Estero for their support during the fieldwork.

References

Ault, S.K., 2007. Pan American Health Organization's Regional Strategic Framework for addressing neglected diseases in neglected populations in Latin America and the Caribbean. *Memórias do Instituto Oswaldo Cruz*, 102 (1), 99–107. Available from: http://www.scielo.br/pdf/mioc/v102s1/cd_14.pdf [Accessed April 2009].

Bastien, J.W., 1998. *The kiss of death. Chagas' disease in the Americas.* Salt Lake City, UT: The University of Utah Press.

Briceño-León, R., 1990. *La casa enferma* [The sick house]. Caracas: Fondo Editorial Acta Científica Venezolana.

Briceño-León, R., 2001. Mud, bugs and community participation. *In*: N. Higginbotham, R. Briceño-León, and N.A. Johnson, eds. *Applying health social science: best practice in the developing world.* London/New York: Zed Books, 226–245.

Bryan, R.T., Balderrama, F., Tonn, R.J., and Dias, J.C., 1994. Community participation in vector control: lessons from Chagas' disease. *American Journal of Tropical Medicine and Hygiene*, 50 (6 Suppl.), 61–71.

Chuit, R., Paulone, I., Wisnivesky-Colli, C., Bo, R., Perez, A.C., Sosa-Stani, S., and Segura, E.L., 1992. Result of a first step toward community-based surveillance of transmission of Chagas' disease with appropriate technology in rural areas. *American Journal for Tropical Medicine and Hygiene*, 46 (4), 444–450.

Cohen, J.M., Wilson, M.L., Cruz-Celis, A., Ordoñez, R., and Ramsey, J.M., 2006. Infestation by *Triatoma pallidipennis* (Hemiptera: Reduviidae: Triatominae) is associated with housing characteristics in rural Mexico. *Journal of Medical Entomology*, 43 (6), 1252–1260.

Crompton, D. and Pearson, M., 2008. *DFID support to the control of neglected tropical diseases: the context* [online]. London: DFID Health Resource Centre. Available from: http://www.dfidhealthrc.org/what_new/DFID%20Support%20to%20the%20control%20of%20NTDs.pdf [Accessed 15 April 2009].

CSDH, 2008. *Closing the gap in a generation: health equity through action on the social determinants of health. Final report of the Commission on Social Determinants of Health.* Geneva: World Health Organization.

Danis-Lozano, R., Rodríguez, M.H., and Hernández-Avila, M., 2002. Gender-related family head schooling and *Aedes aegypti* larval breeding risk in Southern Mexico. *Salud Pública Mexico*, 44, 237–242.

De Maio, F.G., 2007. Health inequalities in Argentina. *Health Sociology Review*, 16 (3–4), 279–291.

De Maio, F.G., Linetzky, B., and Virgolini, M., 2009. An average/deprivation/inequality (ADI) analysis of chronic disease outcomes and risk factors in Argentina. *Population Health Metrics*, 7, 8.

Dias, J.C., 2001. La comunidad y el control de la enfermedad de Chagas: integración, rol, supervisión y evaluación de su participación [Community and Chagas disease control: Integration, role, supervision and evaluation of community participation]. *In*: *Grupo de*

Trabajo OPS en Enfermedad de Chagas. Montevideo: Organización Panamericana de la Salud, 34–50, OPS/HCP/HCT/194.01.

Dias, J.C., 2007. Globalização, iniqüidade e doença de Chagas. *Cadernos de Saúde Pública,* 23 (1), 13–22.

Dias, J.C., Silveira, A.C., and Schofield, C.J., 2002. The impact of Chagas disease control in Latin America – a review. *Memórias do Instituto Oswaldo Cruz,* 97 (5), 603–612.

Espino, F., Koops, V., and Manderson, L., 2004. *Community participation and tropical disease control in resource-poor settings.* TDR/STR/SEB/ST/04.1, Special topics no. 2. Geneva: UNICEF/UNDP/World Bank/WHO – Special Programme for Research and Training in Tropical Diseases (TDR).

Gómez, N., 2004. *Recortes de población en la página del siglo. Lectura de datos censales en Santiago del Estero, 1869–2001.* Primera Parte. La Banda: Universidad Nacional de Santiago del Estero.

Harling, G., Ehrlich, R., and Myer, L., 2008. The social epidemiology of tuberculosis in South Africa: a multilevel analysis. *Social Science and Medicine,* 66 (2), 492–505.

Holveck, J.C., Ehrenberg, J.P., Ault, S.K., Rojas, R., Vasquez, J., Cerqueira, M.T., Ippolito-Shepherd, J., Genovese, M.A., and Periago, M.R., 2007. Prevention, control, and elimination of neglected diseases in the Americas: pathways to integrated, inter-programmatic, inter-sectoral action for health and development. *BioMed Central Public Health,* 7, 6.

Hotez, P.J., Bottazzi, M.E., Franco-Paredes, C., Ault, S.K., and Periago, M.R., 2008. The neglected tropical diseases of Latin America and the Caribbean: a review of disease burden and distribution and a roadmap for control and elimination. *Public Library of Science Neglected Tropical Diseases,* 2 (9), e300.

Hotez, P.J., Molyneux, D.H., Fenwick, A., Kumaresan, J., Ehrlich Sachs, S., Sachs, J.D., and Savioli, L., 2007. Control of neglected tropical diseases [online]. *The New England Journal of Medicine,* 357 (10), 1018–1027. Available from: http://content.nejm.org/cgi/content/full/357/10/1018#R3 [Accessed 15 April 2009].

Hunt, P., 2007. *Neglected diseases: a human rights analysis. Social, economic and behavioural research* [online]. Special topics no. 6. Available from: http://apps.who.int/tdr/publications/tdr-research-publications/neglected-diseases-human-right-analysis/pdf/seb_topic6.pdf [Accessed 15 April 2009].

INDEC, 2001. *Censo nacional de población, hogares y viviendas* [National population, households and housing census]. Buenos Aires: Instituto Nacional de Estadísticas y Censos.

Kahssay, H.M. and Oakley, P., eds., 1999. *Community involvement in health development: a review of the concept and practice.* Geneva: World Health Organization.

Keating, J., MacIntyre, K., Mbogo, C.M., Githure, J.I., and Beier, J.C., 2005. Self-reported malaria and mosquito avoidance in relation to household risk factors in a Kenyan coastal city. *Journal of Biosocial Science,* 37, 761–771.

Llovet, I. and Dinardi, G. 2006. *Decentralization policies and health system reform in Argentina: its impact on Chagas vector prevention and control* [online]. Tenth Global Forum for Health Research, 28 October–3 November, Cairo, EG. Available from: http://www.globalforumhealth.org/filesupld/forum10/F10_finaldocuments/posters/Llovet_Ignacio.pdf [Accessed 15 April 2009].

Llovet, I. and Dinardi, G., 2008. Condiciones sociales y organizativas para la gestión local en salud: re exión a partir de la problemática de la enfermedad de Chagas [Social and organizational conditions for local health management: A re ection based on the challenges posed by Chagas disease]. *In*: M. Chiara, M. Di Virgilio, A. Medina, and M. Miraglia, eds. *Gestión local en salud: conceptos y experiencias.* Buenos Aires: Universidad Nacional de General Sarmiento, 173–182.

Lugones, H.S., 2001. *Enfermedad de Chagas. Diagnóstico de su faz aguda* [Chagas disease. Diagnosis of acute phase]. Santiago del Estero: Ediciones Universidad Católica de Santiago del Estero.

Manderson, L., 1996. *Sickness and the state.* Melbourne and Cambridge: Cambridge University Press.

Manderson, L., Aagaard-Hansen, J., Allotey, P., Gyapong, M., and Sommerfeld, J., 2009. Social research on neglected diseases of poverty: continuing and emerging themes. *Public Library of Science Neglected Tropical Diseases,* 3 (2), e332.

Mathers, C.D., Ezzati, M., and López, A.D., 2007. Measuring the burden of neglected tropical diseases: the global burden of disease framework. *Public Library of Science Neglected Tropical Diseases*, 1 (2), e114.

Mercer, H., 1988. *Aspectos sociológicos del proyecto: estrategia de vigilancia de la transmisión de la enfermedad de Chagas por Atención Primaria de la Salud* [Sociological aspects of the project: Primary Health Care and surveillance strategy for Chagas disease transmission]. Santiago del Estero, AR318.1/WC705/REUN/TERMAS.

Ministerio de Salud, Dirección de Epidemiología, 2002. *Boletín Epidemiológico Nacional.* Buenos Aires: Ministerio de Salud.

Ministerio de Salud, Dirección de Estadísticas e Información en Salud, 2005. *Indicadores Básicos.* Buenos Aires: Ministerio de Salud.

Ministerio de Salud, Dirección de Estadísticas e Información en Salud, 2006. *Indicadores Básicos.* Buenos Aires: Ministerio de Salud.

Moncayo, A., 2003. Chagas disease: current epidemiological trends after the interruption of vectorial and transfusional transmission in the Southern Cone countries. *Memórias do Instituto Oswaldo Cruz*, 98 (5), 577–591.

Morel, C., 2006. Innovation in health and neglected diseases. *Cadernos de Saúde Pública*, 22 (8), 1523.

Morgan, L., 2001. Community participation in health: perpetual allure, persistence challenge. *Health Policy and Planning*, 16 (3), 221–230.

OPS/WHO/NTD/IDM, 2006. *Estimación cuantitativa de la enfermedad de Chagas en las Américas.* Montevideo: Organizatión Panamericana de la Salud, OPS/HDM/CD/425–06.

Prata, A., 2001. Clinical and epidemiological aspects of Chagas disease. *The Lancet Infectious Diseases*, 1 (2), 92–100.

Ramsey, J.M., Alvear, A.L., Ordoñez, R., Muñoz, G., García, A., López, R., and Leyva, R., 2005. Risk factors associated with house infestation by the Chagas disease vector *Triatoma pallidipennis* in Cuernavaca metropolitan area, Mexico. *Medical and Veterinary Entomology*, 19, 219–228.

Segura, E., 2002. El control de la enfermedad de Chagas en la República Argentina [Control of Chagas disease in Argentina]. *In*: C.A. Silveira, ed. *El control de la enfermedad de Chagas en los países del cono sur de América. Historia de una iniciativa internacional* [online]. Organización Panamericana de la Salud. Available from: http://www.paho.org/Spanish/ad/dpc/cd/dch-historia-incosur.pdf [Accessed 15 April 2009].

Segura, E., 2005. *Redes sociales para la vigilancia de la transmisión del Trypanosoma cruzi (Chagas).* Buenos Aires: Ministerio de Salud y Ambiente, Comisión Nacional de Programas de Investigación Sanitaria.

Segura, E.L., Esquivel, M.L., Salomón, O., Gómez, A.O., Sosa Estani, S., Luna, C.A., Tulián, L., Hurvitz, A., Blanco, S., and Andrés, A., 1994. Community participation in the national program for transmission control of Chagas disease. *Medicina.* 54 (5 Pt., 2), 610–611.

Subramanian, S.V., Subramanyam, M.A., Selvaraj, S., and Kawachi, I., 2009. Are self-reports of health and morbidities in developing countries misleading? Evidence from India. *Social Science and Medicine*, 68, 260–265.

TDR/SWG, 2009. *Reporte sobre la enfermedad de Chagas* [Report on Chagas disease]. Ginebra: TDR, Grupo de Trabajo Científico.

Uphoff, N., Esman, M.J., and Krishna, A., 1998. *Reason for success: learning from instructive experiences in rural development.* West Hartfort, CT: Kusmarian Press.

Vaughan, M., 1991. *Curing their ills: colonial power and African illness.* Cambridge: Polity Press.

WHO, 2002. *Control of Chagas disease: second report of the WHO expert committee.* Geneva: WHO, Technical report series 905.

Zaidemberg, M., Spillmann, C., and Carrizo Páez, R., 2004. Control de Chagas en la Argentina. Su evolución. *Revista Argentina de Cardiología*, 72 (5), 375–380.

Chagas disease in non-endemic countries: 'sick immigrant' phobia or a public health concern?

Fernando G. De Maio, Ignacio Llovet and Graciela Dinardi

In recent years, the literature on neglected tropical diseases (NTDs) has advanced in significant ways: there is a renewed sense of urgency in World Health Organization reports, new specialized journals have been launched, and advocacy groups are leveraging social media to gain attention to the burden of NTDs around the world. But as the literature in this field develops, there is a danger of an important split between work that recognizes the profound geopolitical patterning of NTDs, and focuses accordingly on structural factors that lead NTDs to thrive in some areas of the world and not in others; and, alternatively, work that 'securitizes' global health and thereby focuses on the 'risk' posed by NTDs to populations in non-endemic countries. This article examines this schism through the example of Chagas disease.

Introduction

Neglected tropical diseases (NTDs) are a heterogeneous group of parasitic and bacterial diseases that afflict the poorest of the world's poor (Mathers, Ezzati, and Lopez 2007; Hotez 2008). They are thought to affect a total of one billion people worldwide, with most cases occurring in sub-Saharan Africa (WHO 2010). They also continue to exert a heavy toll in parts of Latin America and the Caribbean (Hotez et al. 2008). NTDs differ in their etiology, biological mechanisms, and clinical symptoms, but they share a series of social features; above all, they are bound together by poverty. It is poverty that exposes people to the parasites and bacteria that cause the major NTDs, and it is poverty, along with a lack of global political will, that keeps NTDs under-diagnosed, under-researched, and under-treated.

Indeed, NTDs are a proxy for poverty and disadvantage (Hotez and Ferris 2006); NTDs are prevalent only in settings of poverty and they thrive in zones of military or paramilitary conflict (Beyrer et al. 2007). It is clear that NTDs form a part of a vicious circle: poverty nurtures the risk of contracting an NTD, and NTDs, in turn, severely diminish the economic capacity of individuals and communities, thereby nurturing poverty and inequality. Importantly, this is recognized at the highest levels of global health governance. For example, the WHO proclaims that NTDs 'constitute a serious obstacle to socioeconomic development and quality of life' (2010, 5). Yet, despite this burden, few international resources have been devoted to research on NTD treatment, control, and prevention.

There are signs, however, that NTDs are beginning to receive more attention from global health researchers. The WHO has reenergized this field with several landmark reports in the past few years (WHO 2010, 2012), and advocacy organizations such as 'END7,' which focuses on eliminating ascariasis, hookworm, lymphatic filariasis, onchocerciasis, schistosomiasis, trachoma, and trichuriasis, have gained traction in social media campaigns. Social science engagement with NTDs in English-language journals has also shown promising signs of development in recent years (Spiegel et al. 2010), though much remains to be done. Little has been written from a critical perspective in the social science literature about NTDs, and what exists has not advanced an adequate theorization of the links between global inequities, poverty, structural violence, and NTDs (De Maio forthcoming; Mantilla 2011).

It is important to note that the reference to NTDs as 'neglected' does not imply that they are of secondary importance behind other infectious diseases such as HIV/AIDs, tuberculosis, and malaria – diseases which have gained attention in the Millennium Development Goals. Global health researchers have established that the combined burden of NTDs ranks as high as those of other better-known afflictions in many places, even if their death toll is lower. Rather, '*their neglect reflects their epidemiology*: they are prevalent among the poorest and most marginalized of the world's population' (Manderson et al. 2009, 1; emphasis added). NTDs are burdens of what Beyrer et al. refer to as 'forgotten populations,' emphasizing that because NTDs do not generally affect so-called developed countries, they have been 'largely ignored by medical science' (2007, 619). For Hotez, NTDs are the 'forgotten diseases afflicting forgotten people' (2008, 6). But while forgotten, they are very much real in their impact.

NTDs are estimated to cause more than 500,000 deaths annually – that is, every year NTDs kill as many people as were killed in the 2004 Christmas tsunami (Hotez et al. 2006), but they do not make the news, as their victims are almost entirely confined to the poorest classes in poor countries. NTDs have been largely ignored by the pharmaceutical industry, and until recently, NTDs have also been ignored by social scientists. Recently, however, NTDs have gained more attention from researchers in social science, though funding bias may continue to prohibit the social sciences from playing anything but a marginal role in interdisciplinary teams (Allotey, Reidpath, and Pokhrel 2010; Mantilla 2011; Pokhrel, Reidpath, and Allotey 2011; Reidpath, Allotey, and Pokhrel 2011).

As this field of research develops, it grapples with an important 'framing' debate: do NTDs matter in and of themselves, because they exist, burden poor populations, and could be averted? Or do they matter because they are a threat, can cross national borders and affect non-endemic countries? There is danger of a divide between two kinds of work: one that recognizes the profound geopolitical patterning of NTDs, and focuses accordingly on structural factors that lead NTDs to thrive in some areas of the world. Alternatively, there is work that 'securitizes' global health (Price-Smith 2002; Labonté 2008; Labonté and Gagnon 2010) and thereby narrowly focuses on the 'risk' posed by NTDs to populations in non-endemic countries.

The securitization of global health invokes a state's need to defend itself from external threats (Peterson 2002; Bashford 2006; Aldis 2008). It frames disease as a threat, much like a foreign enemy that must be defeated. In this light, 'global battles' against disease are waged to protect advanced industrialized states from contagion

(Owen and Roberts 2005; Elbe 2010). According to Davies, '... powerful actors still only see a health crisis as worth responding to when it threatens them. Massive national expenditure on disease control can only be justified when governments can draw a link between the threat, infectious disease, and national security' (2010, 22). The problem in all of this, of course, is that a 'securitized' discourse on global health, where disease is primarily seen as a threat to otherwise healthy populations in non-endemic countries, leaves the social conditions wherein disease flourishes intact.

Davies (2010) describes this 'securitized' perspective as the *statist* position (see also Fidler 2005; Maclean 2008; Price-Smith 2009). It has played a fundamental role in global efforts to prevent and control the spread of HIV (Elbe 2006), bringing greater political visibility and funding. Yet as Feldbaum, Lee, and Patel (2006) argue, 'global health works to improve the health of all people within and across states, while the national security field works to protect the people, property, and interests of only one state.' The statist position, based on the notion of securitization, may bring some benefits in terms of disease awareness and research funding, but it comes at a great cost – diverting our attention to the worries of the powerful over the needs of the poor (O'Manique 2006; Brown 2011).

Opposing the statist position, Davies (2010) defines the globalist tradition. This perspective is more strongly tied to the global discourse on human rights and social justice. From this position, disease is seen from the perspective of individuals and marginalized populations, and it need not threaten non-endemic countries to be deemed a political priority. The HIV/AIDS literature is clear that securitization of disease is a nuanced and complex process, bringing benefits and limitations. How this framing process will unfold with NTDs is uncertain – though as examined below, recent attention devoted to the 'globalization' of Chagas to non-endemic countries indicates that the statist perspective may be growing in importance.

Chagas disease

Chagas disease is Latin America's most important parasitic disease (WHO 2010; Llovet, Dinardi, and De Maio 2011). It is spread primarily by a 'kissing bug'; these blood-sucking *triatomine* insects live in crevices of the walls and roofs of very poor homes; they thrive in the crooks and gaps left in mud-thatch construction and in walls made of precarious building materials. When they bite they defecate into the bite wound, and in doing so can transmit a parasite (*Trypanosoma cruzi; T. cruzi*) into its victim, leading to Chagas disease. Chagas infection is followed by two phases: acute and chronic. The acute phase can last from 4–8 weeks, and is characterized by fever, swollen lymph glands, and often, inflammation at the biting site. Up to 40% of infected people develop chronic Chagas disease (Reithinger et al. 2009), which is characterized by cardiac and gastrointestinal complications. If left untreated, these can be fatal. In disease endemic areas like Bolivia, Paraguay, and northern Argentina, Chagas is the leading factor in cardiovascular deaths (Reithinger et al. 2009). There is concern in the literature; however, over how difficult it is to isolate the cardiovascular effects of *T. cruzi* seropositivity from the pathogenic effects of poverty (Linetzky et al., 2012). Almost a third of patients are estimated to develop Chagas-related heart damage, and 10% to develop damage to the oesophagus, colon, or nervous system (or a combination of these), typically in the late chronic phase of the disease (WHO 2010).

It is a quintessential disease of poverty – one that poor peasants are at most risk of contracting, one that is largely undiagnosed, and one that has never been a priority for

for-profit pharmaceutical research (only two pharmacological interventions for Chagas exist, and both are over 30 years old, with limited effectiveness, toxic side effects, and complicated dosing regimens). This reflects a true 'market failure,' whereby the lives of the poor are deemed to be of little value; the development of new vaccines or treatments failing contemporary judgments of 'cost-effectiveness' (Trouiller et al. 2002). Unique to the Americas, Chagas generates an estimated burden of 426,000 DALYs every year (WHO 2010). It is almost entirely associated with poor quality housing in rural settings.

An estimated 7–8 million people are thought to be infected in the region of the Americas (with some estimates more in the 10–20 million range – there is a lot of imprecision in these estimates), with most of these cases being asymptomatic and undiagnosed (Reithinger et al. 2009). Endemic areas exist in 21 countries of Latin America (Dias 2009). Argentina, Brazil, and Mexico are thought to have the largest number of cases of *T. cruzi* infection, at more than one million cases in each country (Franco-Paredes, Bottazzi, and Hotez 2009; WHO 2010). But Bolivia has the highest rate of *T. cruzi* infection in the world, with an estimated 6% of the overall population infected (WHO 2010). Some surveys of pregnant women and blood donors in hyperendemic communities reach prevalence rates of 30–40% in that country (Breniere et al. 2002; Pirard et al. 2005). Despite these high figures, few NGOs work explicitly with Chagas patients, and the END7 campaign – which has gained traction in social media to generate public awareness of NTDs – does not include Chagas in its focus.

Vector transmission is the most important way of spreading Chagas disease – but it can also be spread through transfusions with infected blood and it can also be passed from mother to fetus through the placenta (Barona-Vilar et al. 2012; Carlier et al. 2011). Improved blood donation screening mechanisms in Latin America have diminished disease transmission as a result of transfusion (WHO 2010). Whereas in 1990, only Argentina, Honduras, Uruguay, and Venezuela performed serological screening of all blood donors for *T. cruzi*, the list of countries which screen all donors has now risen to 8, including Brazil, the most populous country in the region. Four other countries now screen 99% of blood donors (Schmunis 2007). However, that is not to say that this has resulted in diminished attention to the prospect of *T. cruzi* transmission through blood transfusion and/or organ transplantation. A new wave of articles and WHO reports raise the spectre of a 'globalised Chagas,' emphasizing the global risk of Chagas in non-endemic countries.

The spectre of a 'Globalized' chagas

Chagas disease has been detected in non-endemic countries where vector transmission does not exist (due either to climate and/or housing infrastructure which is unsuitable for triatomine insects). There, migrants have brought *T. cruzi* infection with them and pose a danger of transmitting the parasite into the blood supply, and congenital transmission is also a possibility among migrants groups. Increased recognition of this epidemiological patterning may lead to improved resources for affected groups – but it may also lead to a further stigmatization of NTDs like Chagas and a backlash reminiscent of the 'sick immigrant' paradigm (Beiser 2005; De Maio 2010).

Schmunis' (2007) analysis of Chagas spreading along immigration routes is an important article in this area. He plotted legal and undocumented migration flows from Latin America to the global north to estimate the global epidemiology of Chagas in non-endemic countries. Schmunis gathered information on the number of immigrants, both documented and undocumented, from national statistical agencies in receiving countries; he then took into account the prevalence of infection in the country of origin, and estimated the size of the population in each country that may be expected to have *T. cruzi* in their blood. He estimates that the number of infected migrants is in the thousands for Australia, Canada, and Spain, and in the tens or even hundreds of thousands in the USA. Some work now cites that up to a million people may carry Chagas in the USA (Hotez et al. 2012), although these are only estimates; no population registers of Chagas-infected people exist or are technically/ethically viable. Supporting Schmunis' argument, a new wave of empirical studies has examined Chagas seropositivity among immigrants. For example, a study of blood donors in New York City found a 'persistent and possibly increasing population of patients with Chagas infection,' associating this prevalence with foreign born people, mainly Salvadorian and Mexican (Zaniello et al. 2012). Another study at a health center in Barcelona found an even larger prevalence than in the New York study, mainly affecting Bolivian born people (Roca et al. 2011). These studies support Schmunis' affirmation: 'there is ample evidence that non endemic countries harbor a population of individuals infected with *T. cruzi*, and that, sooner or later, nations should have to confront the prevention of transfusion or organ-acquired infection, as well as secondary prevention of congenital infection' (2007, 79). At the same time, Schmunis thoughtfully raises a warning of possible unintended consequence of this line of analysis, urging that legislation be developed to protect immigrants from discrimination over their *potential* infection.

The spectre of a globalized Chagas has also been raised in other studies. For example Perez De Ayala et al. (2009) document cases of chagasic cardiomyopathy in immigrants from Latin America in Spain and Jackson et al. (2009) describe congenital transmission of Chagas among Latin American immigrants in Switzerland. Studies like this appropriately signal the need for public health efforts against Chagas disease in non-endemic countries; this could be aimed at raising awareness among physicians about the disease, for example. And new procedures could be implemented to ensure that *T. cruzi*-infected blood is not accepted by blood banks. Along these lines, the US Food and Drug Administration recently issued guidance to blood banks in the USA for screening of Chagas (Ribeiro et al. 2009).

Most recently, Hotez et al. received widespread media coverage for their editorial dubbing Chagas the 'new' HIV/AIDS of the Americas (see Hotez et al. 2012), and popular media reports of the editorial emphasized the 'new' threat posed by the disease to the US population (for e.g. see Jauregui 2012; Mcneil 2012). These reports noted the burden of Chagas disease in Latin America, but overwhelmingly focused on the alarmist threat that the disease was something that would spread to the USA. The way in which the media sensationalized the Hotez et al. editorial is indicative of securitization, with Chagas coming to matter only when it was re-branded as a threat to populations in industrialized countries. At a time when the USA is experiencing profound battles over access to health care services, the notion that large numbers of immigrants bring an additional health burden to the native-born population may generate increased xenophobia and discrimination.

A focus on Chagas disease in non-endemic countries may also take our attention away from the more important picture, shifting our focus from the poor of the global south to the 'worried well' of the global north. Chagas disease in non-endemic countries is part of 'global health,' certainly – but the shift in emphasis and gaze distracts us from the real victims of NTDs, the poorest of the poor, and harkens back to images of the 'sick immigrant' paradigm, where immigrants are to be feared and immigration to be controlled if disease is not to run rampant in otherwise 'clean' places (Beiser 2005; De Maio 2010).

From the globalist perspective, Chagas disease is not important just because it may spread to non-endemic countries, tainting their blood supplies and requiring specialized costly treatments for those affected, but because it continues to burden poor populations in the global south, causing unnecessary morbidity and premature mortality. From this perspective, NTDs need not threaten the industrialized countries to be deemed a priority. One of the challenges in contemporary global health research is to strengthen the globalist position on NTDs; to make it – rather than the statist perspective – the normative lens. Overcoming the reactionary and defensive characteristics of statist thinking in global health is a tremendous challenge, but one that can be met, as evidenced by the work of non-government organizations such as Partners in Health and *Médecins sans Frontiéres*.

At the same time, advancing the globalist perspective in NTD research will necessitate a critical reappraisal of possible solutions. Chagas disease offers a particularly strong rebuke to claims that pharmaceutical or biochemical solutions are sufficient. Vector control through insecticide spraying – while effective in the short term – raises long-term questions, beginning with the health effects of exposing populations and the environment to toxins, as well as the very real threat of vectors developing insecticide resistance, signs of which have already been documented (Dias, Prata, and Correia 2008). Instead of relying on vector control through the spraying of insecticides, a structural approach to reducing the burden of Chagas disease in the Americas would focus on improving the housing stock of poor populations, recognizing that the bug vectors thrive in the building materials use by rural peasants throughout the region (WHO 2012). A shift from biomedical to structural solutions may very well challenge contemporary funding arrangements, based on the priorities and interests of major global philanthropic organizations as well as national funders like the Canadian Institutes for Health Research and the US National Institutes of Health. However, such a shift could signal a much needed return to the progressive history of public health – a profession which at its best engages with and challenges structural arrangements that cause harm to populations (Navarro 2008; Raphael 2011; White 2012).

Conclusion

Chagas disease is unique among the NTDs for its ability to be framed as a threat under a 'securitized' global health paradigm. Other NTDs, including schistosomiasis and lymphatic filariasis, have far more limited geographic scope, and to the extent that global health research is guided by issues of securitization, these and other NTDs will continue to afflict the poorest of the poor without ever becoming a priority. They will remain the forgotten diseases of forgotten people. Alternatively, social scientists may yet contribute to the NTD literature by examining the structural roots of NTD epidemiology. NTDs thrive on poverty, on political marginalization and neglect, on unmet basic needs. Global health researchers have done much to map out the distribution of NTDs, and we now know more than ever before about their prevalence and incidence. And effective policies – rooted, above all, in the improvements of living conditions for the poorest of the poor – may yet be developed. It is our challenge to raise awareness of NTDs such as Chagas while at the same time supporting a globalist position on health; diseases like Chagas matter, not just when they become a threat to populations in industrialized countries, but rather, because they are an avoidable, unnecessary, and unfair component of global health inequality.

References

Aldis, W. 2008. "Health Security as a Public Health Concept: A Critical Analysis." *Health Policy and Planning* 23 (6): 369–375.

Allotey, P., D. D. Reidpath, and S. Pokhrel. 2010. "Social Sciences Research in Neglected Tropical Diseases 1: The Ongoing Neglect in the Neglected Tropical Diseases." *Health Research Policy and Systems* 8 (32). http://www.health-policy-systems.com/content/pdf/1478-4505-8-32.pdf

Barona-Vilar, C., M. J. Gimenez-Marti, T. Fraile, C. Gonzalez-Steinbauer, C. Parada, A. Gil-Brusola, D. Bravo, et al. 2012. "Prevalence of *Trypanosoma cruzi* Infection in Pregnant Latin American Women and Congenital Transmission Rate in a Non-endemic Area: The Experience of the Valencian Health Programme (Spain)." *Epidemiology and Infection* 10 (10): 1896–1903.

Bashford, A., ed. 2006. *Medicine at the Border: Disease, Globalization and Security, 1850 to the Present*. Basingstoke: Palgrave Macmillan.

Beiser, M. 2005. "The Health of Immigrants and Refugees in Canada." *Canadian Journal of Public Health* 96 (Suppl 2): S30–S44.

Beyrer, C., J. C. Villar, V. Suwanvanichkij, S. Singh, S. D. Baral, and E. J. Mills. 2007. "Neglected Diseases, Civil Conflicts, and the Right to Health." *Lancet* 370 (9587): 619–627.

Breniere, S. F., M. F. Bosseno, F. Noireau, N. Yacsik, P. Liegeard, C. Aznar, and M. Hontebeyrie. 2002. "Integrate Study of a Bolivian Population Infected by *Trypanosoma cruzi*, the Agent of Chagas Disease." *Memórias do Instituto Oswaldo Cruz* 97 (3): 289–295.

Brown, T. 2011. "'Vulnerability is Universal': Considering the Place of 'Security' and 'Vulnerability' within Contemporary Global Health Discourse." *Social Science & Medicine* 72 (3): 319–326.

Carlier, Y., F. Torrico, S. Sosa-Estani, G. Russomando, A. Luquetti, H. Freilij, and P. Albajar Vinas. 2011. "Congenital Chagas Disease: Recommendations for Diagnosis, Treatment and Control of Newborns, Siblings and Pregnant Women." *PLoS Neglected Tropical Diseases* 5 (10): e1250.

Davies, S. E. 2010. *Global Politics of Health*. Cambridge: Polity Press.

De Maio, F. G. Forthcoming. *Global Health Inequities: A Sociological Perspective*. Basignstoke: Palgrave Macmillan.

De Maio, F. G. 2010. "Immigration as Pathogenic: A Systematic Review of the Health of Immigrants to Canada." *International Journal for Equity in Health* 9 (27). http://www.ncbi.nlm.nih.gov/pmc/articles/PMC2999602/pdf/1475-9276-9-27.pdf

Dias, J. C. 2009. "Elimination of Chagas Disease Transmission: Perspectives." *Memórias do Instituto Oswaldo Cruz* 104 (Suppl 1): 41–45.

Dias, J. C., A. Prata, and D. Correia. 2008. "Problems and Perspectives for Chagas Disease Control: In Search of a Realistic Analysis." *Revista da Sociedade Brasileira de Medicina Tropical* 41 (2): 193–196.

Elbe, S. 2006. "Should HIV/AIDS Be Securitized? The Ethical Dilemma of Linking HIV/AIDS and Security." *International Studies Quarterly* 50 (1): 119–144.

Elbe, S. 2010. *Security and Global Health*. Cambridge: Polity.

Feldbaum, H., K. Lee, and P. Patel. 2006. "The National Security Implications of HIV/AIDS." *PLoS Medicine* 3 (6): e171.

Fidler, D. P. 2005. "Health as Foreign Policy: Between Principle and Power." *Whitehead Journal of Diplomacy and International Relations* 6 (2): 179–194.

Franco-Paredes, C., M. E. Bottazzi, and P. J. Hotez. 2009. "The Unfinished Public Health Agenda of Chagas Disease in the Era of Globalization." *PLoS Neglected Tropical Diseases* 3 (7): e470.

Hotez, P. J. 2008. *Forgotten People, Forgotten Diseases: The Neglected Tropical Diseases and their Impact on Global Health and Developmen*. Washington, DC: ASM Press.

Hotez, P. J., M. E. Bottazzi, C. Franco-Paredes, S. K. Ault, and M. R. Periago. 2008. "The Neglected Tropical Diseases of Latin America and the Caribbean: A Review of Disease Burden and Distribution and a Roadmap for Control and Elimination." *PLoS Neglected Tropical Diseases* 2 (9): e300.

Hotez, P. J., E. Dumonteil, L. Woc-Colburn, J. A. Serpa, S. Bezek, M. S. Edwards, C. J. Hallmark, L. W. Musselwhite, B. J. Flink, and M. E. Bottazzi. 2012. "Chagas Disease: 'The New HIV/AIDS of the Americas'." *PLoS Neglected Tropical Diseases* 6 (5): e1498.

Hotez, P. J., and M. T. Ferris. 2006. "The Antipoverty Vaccines." *Vaccine* 24 (31–32): 5787–5799.

Hotez, P. J., E. A. Ottesen, A. Fenwick, and D. Molyneux. 2006. "The Neglected Tropical Diseases: The Ancient Afflictions of Stigma and Poverty and the Prospects for their Control and Elimination." In *Hot Topics in Infection and Immunity in Children*, edited by A. J. Pollard and A. Finn, 23–33. New York: Springer.

Jackson, Y., C. Myers, A. Diana, H. P. Marti, H. Wolff, F. Chappuis, L. Loutan, and A. Gervaix. 2009. "Congenital Transmission of Chagas Disease in Latin American Immigrants in Switzerland." *Emerging Infectious Diseases* 15 (4): 601–603.

Jauregui, A. 2012. "Chagas Disease, Tropical Insect-bore Illness, may be 'New HIV/AIDS of the Americas'." *Huffington Post*, May 30.

Labonté, R. 2008. "Global Health in Public Policy: Finding the Right Frame?" *Critical Public Health* 18 (4): 467–482.

Labonté, R., and M. L. Gagnon. 2010. "Framing Health and Foreign Policy: Lessons for Global Health Diplomacy." *Globalization and Health* 6 (14).

Linetzky, B., J. Konfino, N. Castellana, F.G. De Maio, M.C. Bahit, A. Orlandini, and R. Diaz. 2012. "Risk of Cardiovascular Events Associated with Positive Serology for Chagas: A Systematic Review." *International Journal of Epidemiology*. 41 (5): 1356–1366.

Llovet, I., G. Dinardi, and F. G. De Maio. 2011. "Mitigating Social and Health Inequities: Community Participation and Chagas Disease in Rural Argentina." *Global Public Health* 6 (4): 371–384.

Maclean, S. J. 2008. "Microbes, Mad Cows and Militaries: Exploring the Links between Health and Security." *Security Dialogue* 39 (5): 475–494.

Manderson, L., J. Aagaard-Hansen, P. Allotey, M. Gyapong, and J. Sommerfeld. 2009. "Social Research on Neglected Diseases of Poverty: Continuing and Emerging Themes." *PLoS Neglected Tropical Diseases* 3 (2): e332.

Mantilla, B. 2011. "Invisible Plagues, Invisible Voices: A Critical Discourse Analysis of Neglected Tropical Diseases." *Social Medicine* 6 (3): 118–127.

Mathers, C. D., M. Ezzati, and A. D. Lopez. 2007. "Measuring the Burden of Neglected Tropical Diseases: The Global Burden of Disease Framework." *PLoS Neglected Tropical Diseases* 1 (2): e114.

Mcneil, D. G. 2012. "Stubborn Infection, Spread by Insects, is Called 'the New AIDS of the Americas'." *New York Times*, May 28.

Navarro, V. 2008. "Politics and Health: A Neglected Area of Research." *European Journal of Public Health* 18 (4): 354–355.

O'Manique, C. 2006. "The "Securitisation" of HIV/AIDS in Sub-Saharan Africa: A Critical Feminist Lens." In *A Decade of Human Security: Global Governance and the New Multilateralisms*, edited by Sandra J. Maclean, David R. Black, and Timothy M. Shaw, 168–176. Aldershot: Ashgate.

Owen, J. W., and O. Roberts. 2005. "Globalization, Health and Foreign Policy: Emerging Linkages and Interests." *Globalization and Health* 1 (12). http://www.globalizationandhealth.com/content/1/1/12

Perez De Ayala, A., J. A. Perez-Molina, F. Norman, and R. Lopez-Velez. 2009. "Chagasic Cardiomyopathy in Immigrants from Latin America to Spain." *Emerging Infectious Diseases* 15 (4): 607–608.

Peterson, S. 2002. "Epidemic Disease and National Security." *Security Studies* 12 (2): 43–81.

Pirard, M., N. Iihoshi, M. Boelaert, P. Basanta, F. Lopez, and P. Van Der Stuyft. 2005. "The Validity of Serologic Tests for *Trypanosoma cruzi* and the Effectiveness of Transfusional Screening Strategies in a Hyperendemic Region." *Transfusion* 45 (4): 554–561.

Pokhrel, S., D. Reidpath, and P. Allotey. 2011. "Social Sciences Research in Neglected Tropical Diseases 3: Investment in Social Science Research in Neglected Diseases of Poverty: A Case Study of Bill and Melinda Gates Foundation." *Health Research Policy and Systems* 9 (2). http://www.health-policy-systems.com/content/pdf/1478-4505-9-1.pdf

Price-Smith, A. T. 2002. *The Health of Nations: Infectious Disease, Environmental Change, and their Effects on National Security and Development.* Cambridge, MA: MIT Press.

Price-Smith, A. T. 2009. *Contagion and Chaos: Disease, Ecology, and National Security in the Era of Globalization.* Cambridge, MA: The MIT Press.

Raphael, D. 2011. "A Discourse Analysis of the Social Determinants of Health." *Critical Public Health* 21 (2): 221–236.

Reidpath, D. D., P. Allotey, and S. Pokhrel. 2011. "Social Sciences Research in Neglected Tropical Diseases 2: A Bibliographic Analysis." *Health Research Policy and Systems* 9 (1). http://www.health-policy-systems.com/content/pdf/1478-4505-9-1.pdf

Reithinger, R., R. L. Tarleton, J. A. Urbina, U. Kitron, and R. E. Gurtler. 2009. "Eliminating Chagas Disease: Challenges and a Roadmap." *British Medical Journal* 338: 1044–1046. http://www.bmj.com/highwire/section-pdf/8846/7/1

Ribeiro, I., A. M. Sevcsik, F. Alves, G. Diap, R. Don, M. O. Harhay, S. Chang, and B. Pecoul. 2009. "New, Improved Treatments for Chagas Disease: From the R&D Pipeline to the Patients." *PLoS Neglected Tropical Diseases* 3 (7): e484.

Roca, C., M. J. Pinazo, P. Lopez-Chejade, J. Bayo, E. Posada, J. Lopez-Solana, M. Gallego, M. Portus, and J. Gascon. 2011. "Chagas Disease among the Latin American Adult Population Attending in a Primary Care Center in Barcelona, Spain." *PLoS Neglected Tropical Diseases* 5 (4): e1135.

Schmunis, G. A. 2007. "Epidemiology of Chagas Disease in Non-endemic Countries: The Role of International Migration." *Memórias do Instituto Oswaldo Cruz* 102 (Suppl 1): 75–85.

Spiegel, J. M., S. Dharamsi, K. M. Wasan, A. Yassi, B. Singer, P. J. Hotez, C. Hanson, and D. A. Bundy. 2010. "Which New Approaches to Tackling Neglected Tropical Diseases Show Promise?" *PLoS Medicine* 7 (5): e1000255.

Trouiller, P., P. Olliaro, E. Torreele, J. Orbinski, R. Laing, and N. Ford. 2002. "Drug Development for Neglected Diseases: A Deficient Market and a Public-Health Policy Failure." *Lancet* 359 (9324): 2188–2194.

White, S. K. 2012. "Public Health at a Crossroads: Assessing Teaching on Economic Globalization as a Social Determinant of Health." *Critical Public Health* 22 (3): 281–295.

WHO (World Health Organization). 2010. *Working to Overcome the Global Impact of Neglected Tropical Diseases: First WHO Report on Neglected Tropical Diseases.* Geneva: World Health Organization.

WHO (World Health Organization). 2012. *Accelerating Work to Overcome the Global Impact of Neglected Tropical Diseases: A Roadmap for Implementation.* Geneva: World Health Organization.

Zaniello, B. A., D. A. Kessler, K. M. Vine, K. M. Grima, and S. A. Weisenberg. 2012. "Seroprevalence of Chagas Infection in the Donor Population." *PLoS Neglected Tropical Diseases* 6 (7): e1771.

Extending the income inequality hypothesis: Ecological results from the 2005 and 2009 Argentine National Risk Factor Surveys

Fernando G. De Maio, Bruno Linetzky, Daniel Ferrante and
Nancy L. Fleischer

A consensus on income inequality as a social determinant of health is yet to be reached. In particular, we know little about the cross-sectional versus lagged effect of inequality and the robustness of the relationship to indicators that are sensitive to varying parts of the income spectrum. We test these issues with data from Argentina's 2005 and 2009 National Risk Factor Surveys. Inequality was operationalised at the provincial level with the Gini coefficient and the Generalised Entropy (GE) index. Population health was defined as the age-standardised percentage of adults with poor/fair self-rated health by province. Our cross-sectional results indicate a significant relationship between inequality (Gini) and poor health ($r = 0.58$, $p < 0.01$) in 2005. Using the GE index, a gradient pattern emerges in the correlation, and the r values increase as the index becomes sensitive to the top of the distribution. The relationship between 2005 inequality and 2009 health displays a similar pattern, but with generally smaller correlations than the 2005 cross-sectional results. Further advances in the income inequality and health literature require new theoretical models to account for how inequalities in different parts of the income spectrum may influence population health in different ways.

Introduction

The income inequality hypothesis has been examined through a variety of statistical approaches – from ecological to multi-level – and through both positivist and critical realist epistemologies (Coburn 2004, Wilkinson and Pickett 2008, 2009b, De Maio 2010). Despite a large empirical and theoretical literature (Wilkinson and Pickett 2009a, De Maio 2012), little agreement exists on its overall validity. Researchers have raised questions about the geographical level in which the hypothesis should be tested, the regions in the world where the hypothesis might apply (Lynch *et al.* 2003, 2004, Subramanian and Kawachi 2003) and which health indicators should be used (De Maio 2007a, 2008).

Lending credence to the idea of a 'threshold' effect, wherein income inequality has a detectable effect on health but only at or above a certain level of inequality, significant effects have been detected in the relatively unequal countries of China (Pei and Rodriguez 2006), Italy (De Vogli *et al.* 2005), Brazil (Cavalini and de Leon 2008), Chile (Subramanian *et al.* 2003) and Argentina (De Maio 2008). This contrasts with null findings from the relatively equal areas/countries of Scandinavia (Böckerman *et al.* 2009), Germany (Breckenkamp *et al.* 2007), Denmark (Osler *et al.* 2002, 2003), Canada (Veenstra 2002, Auger *et al.* 2009) and Japan (Shibuya *et al.* 2002). Recently, Dunn *et al.* (2007) have argued that instead of dismissing the income inequality hypothesis, because it does not appear to hold true in all cases under all conditions, research should focus on the particular question of 'under what conditions does the relationship between income inequality and population health hold?'.

Most ecological analyses of the income inequality hypothesis have been static in the sense that they have analysed data from one particular point in time. This is partly attributable to the relative paucity of historical data on income inequality (Leigh and Jencks 2007), particularly at levels of geography lower than the nation state. However, there is reason to believe that the health effect of income inequality may lag, and income inequality in year 1 may influence health in year $1 + n$ (Laporte and Ferguson 2003, Lynch *et al.* 2005, Leigh and Jencks 2007), with some authors suggesting that a lag of up to 15 years may be appropriate (Blakely *et al.* 2000). This is particularly relevant for the neo-material pathway, which asserts that income inequality is associated with systematic underinvestment in social infrastructure (e.g., education, health services, transportation, the availability of nutritious food, occupational health controls and housing) (Kahn *et al.* 2000). In effect, the neo-material explanation sees income inequality as a result of historical, cultural, political and economic processes that manifest themselves by influencing public infrastructure. From this perspective, it is plausible to posit that it may take years for inequality to 'get under the skin'. The psychosocial pathway, which sees a more direct link between inequality and health, is also consistent with the idea of a lagged effect. From this perspective, inequality is experienced as a stress-inducing stimulus activating both the allostatic load model (McEwen 1998) and the 'fight or flight' syndrome (Brunner 1997, Wilkinson 2000). A lagged effect is also compatible with this perspective, as the health effects of exposure to high inequality may take years to manifest in the body. More detailed accounts of the neo-material and psychosocial perspectives are offered by Kawachi *et al.* (1999) and De Maio (2010).

Our study uses new nationally representative survey data of 2005 and 2009 from Argentina to examine the ecological relationship between income inequality and population health with a 4-year time lag. This builds directly from the results of previous studies that suggest that an important place to examine the health effects of income inequality is the high-inequality countries of Latin America (Subramanian *et al.* 2003). Countries like Argentina have an epidemiological profile not unlike the countries of the Organization for Economic Co-Operation and Development (OECD), where the majority of studies of the income inequality hypothesis have been carried out. In Argentina, the leading causes of death are non-communicable diseases (Ferrante 2006), with cardiovascular diseases and cancers exerting the heaviest burdens. This 'post-transition' epidemiological profile is at the crux of Wilkinson's writings on the income inequality model and makes Argentina a relevant country in which to study the health effects of inequality.

Our work builds on the notion that income inequality may be operationalised using a number of different approaches (Jenkins 1991, De Maio 2007b, Chakravarty

2009). The most common approach has been to use the Gini coefficient. Building from an influential study by Kawachi and Kennedy (1997), which tested the robustness of the hypothesis using ecological data from US states and found a high correlation among income inequality measures and consistent correlations between income inequality indicators and mortality rates, researchers in this area have tended to ignore the subtleties that may be detected using myriad inequality indicators. The Gini coefficient has emerged as the default income inequality measure, and while this is appropriate in many cases, it does involve the loss of important information; much might be learned by examining how the income inequality–population health relationship is influenced by the sensitivity of the inequality indictor to inequalities in different parts of the income spectrum.

The Gini coefficient is incapable of differentiating different kinds of inequalities. Lorenz curves may intersect, reflecting differing patterns of income distribution, nevertheless resulting in very similar Gini coefficient values (Atkinson 1975, Cowell 1995). This troubling property of the Lorenz framework complicates comparisons of Gini coefficient values and may confound tests of the income inequality hypothesis. In addition, it is known that the Gini coefficient is most sensitive to inequalities in the middle part of the income spectrum (Hey and Lambert 1980, Ellison 2002). This may be appropriate in many studies, but in some cases, researchers will have valid reasons to emphasise income gaps in the top or bottom of the spectrum (Wen *et al.* 2003). For example, Weich *et al.* (2002), in their study of income inequality and self-rated health using the British Household Panel Survey, found important differences between the Gini coefficient and the Generalised Entropy (GE) index. They observed that regional income inequality, operationalised using the Gini coefficient, was significantly associated with poor health among respondents from low income groups, but that this relationship was not significant for GE indicators sensitive to inequalities at the top or bottom of the income spectrum. The extent to which the Gini coefficient differs from other measures of income distribution can therefore be an important source of insight into the health effects of income inequality.

Building from this existing body of literature, the present study tests two methodological aspects: (1) the cross-sectional versus lagged effect of income inequality and (2) the robustness of the income inequality–population health relationship to inequality indicators that are sensitive to inequalities in different parts of the income spectrum.

Methods

Data from Argentina's 2005 and 2009 National Risk Factor Surveys (*Encuesta Nacional de Factores de Riesgo* – ENFR) are used in these analyses. Both are nationally and provincially representative surveys. The 2005 ENFR has a sample size of 41,392 adults and a response rate of 86.7% (Ferrante and Virgolini 2007), whereas the 2009 ENFR has a sample size of 34,732 and a response rate of 79.8% (MSAL 2011). Both surveys were carried out by Argentina's Ministry of Health in cooperation with the *Instituto Nacional de Estadística y Censos* (INDEC; National Institute of Statistics and Census) and provincial authorities. Methodological features of the ENFR have been presented in previous reports (Ferrante and Virgolini 2007, Fleischer *et al.* 2008, De Maio *et al.* 2009).

Five different income inequality indexes are used in this study: the Gini coefficient and four categories of the GE Index: GE(-1), GE(0), GE(1) and GE(2), with the latter also known in the economics literature as Theil's measure. The Gini coefficient is derived from the Lorenz curve of the plot of cumulative percentage of the population by socio-economic status and cumulative percentage of total income; a Gini coefficient of 0 reflects a perfectly equal society in which all income is shared equally, and a Gini coefficient of 1 represents a perfectly unequal society wherein all income is earned by one individual. The Gini coefficient's main weakness as a measure of income distribution is that it is incapable of differentiating different kinds of inequalities; Lorenz curves may intersect (reflecting differing patterns of income distribution) but may nevertheless result in the same Gini coefficient value.

In contrast, the GE index incorporates a sensitivity parameter to help differentiate different patterns of inequality: the more positive α is (the sensitivity parameter: -1, 0, 1, or 2), the more sensitive GE(α) is to inequalities at the top of the income distribution, whereas lower values of α indicate that the GE index is sensitive to differences at the bottom of the distribution (Jenkins 1999). The idea behind the sensitivity parameter is that inequality can grow because of income gaps in the middle of the spectrum (and the Gini coefficient is most sensitive to this) as well as income gaps in the top (richest) and bottom (poorest) tails of the distribution. These are qualitatively different patterns of inequality and something that the Gini coefficient cannot detect. The GE index is therefore a valuable tool that allows the measurement of qualitatively different patterns of inequality. Regardless of the choice of α, the GE index produces results that can range from 0 to ∞, with 0 being a state of equal distribution and values greater than 0 representing increasing levels of inequality.

Household income data were available in the 2005 ENFR dataset in 19 categories, with 100 peso intervals for incomes below 1,000 pesos, 250 peso intervals for incomes between 1,000 and 2,000 and 1,000 peso intervals for incomes between 2,000 and 5,000 pesos. The last category included incomes of more than 5,000 pesos per month, with no upper bound. Following De Vaus (2002), we assigned the mid-point value to each category (e.g., respondents with household income of 301–400 pesos were coded as having 350 pesos). Given that the last category had no upper bound, we followed a conservative strategy of coding 5,000 and above as 5,500.

Income inequality indices were generated using Stata's ineqdeco programme (Jenkins 1999). Gini estimates from the ENFR were compared to estimates derived using Argentina's *Encuesta Permanente de Hogares* (EPH), a long-running survey of income and labour in the country. National and sub-national levels of inequality were similar in both datasets (results not shown). The EPH, however, is not designed for provincial-level analysis and we therefore used the inequality estimates from the ENFR itself. Self-rated health, an indicator derived from the SF-36 questionnaire, was measured using a five-point scale: excellent, very good, good, fair or poor. Following conventional practice, this variable was recoded as a binary outcome (excellent, very good, or good versus fair or poor).

Along with our income inequality indices, we considered associations between poor health and provincial poverty, as indicated by the percentage of homes in a province with at least one unmet basic need (UBN). UBN is defined in the 2005 ENFR by the following household characteristics: (1) a lack sufficient dwelling space (defined as more than 3 people per room), (2) inadequate housing/building material (e.g., dirt floor), (3) a lack of proper sanitary conditions (e.g., a working toilet) or (4) the presence of school-age children (6–12 years) who are not enrolled in school. UBN is a widely used measure of absolute poverty in Argentina (Javier *et al.* 1995, INDEC 2003, Marín *et al.* 2008) and other countries in Latin America (Peña *et al.* 2000, Montilva *et al.* 2003).

Both the 2005 and 2009 ENFR were designed to be representative at the national and provincial levels. We aggregated the micro data to the level of the province, creating provincial-level measures of income inequality and self-rated health (age standardised percentage in poor/fair health). This results in an *N* of 24 ecological units (23 provinces and the Federal District of Buenos Aires). Adjustment by age was done through direct standardisation using the national standard population (year 2000) as a reference. The data were analysed using Pearson correlation coefficients. Scatterplots of all correlations were examined for non-linear associations. Following previous analyses of this type, correlations were weighted by provincial population (Ross *et al.* 2000, De Maio 2008). All analyses were carried out using Stata 11. Stata's survey analysis feature was used to calculate the regional aggregates.

Results

Summary univariate statistics for provincial-level income inequality and self-rated health are presented in Table 1. Among the income inequality indicators, GE(-1) and GE(2) display the most variation, in terms of range and standard deviation.

The relationship between income inequality in 2005, operationalised as the Gini coefficient, and the percentage of adults in a province with poor/fair health in that year is positive ($r = 0.58$, $p < 0.01$; see Figure 1). When income inequality is operationalised with the GE index, a gradient pattern emerges in the coefficients, and the *r* values increase as the GE index becomes more and more sensitive to inequalities at the top of the income distribution (Table 2). The correlation is strongest with GE(2), with a correlation of 0.75 ($p < 0.01$). However, when the GE index is particularly sensitive to inequalities at the bottom of the income distribution

Table 1. Summaries of provincial-level indicators.

	Mean	Minimum	Maximum	Standard deviation
Income inequality – 2005				
Gini	0.42	0.35	0.47	0.02
GE(-1)	0.46	0.33	0.57	0.04
GE(0)	0.31	0.24	0.39	0.03
GE(1)	0.29	0.20	0.40	0.03
GE(2)	0.37	0.21	0.60	0.06
Unmet basic needs (UBN,%)	17.8	4.8	41.7	7.9
% with poor/fair self-rated health[a]				
2005	20.6	14.0	37.7	5.1
2009	19.7	13.7	29.0	4.5

Note: [a]Age standardised.

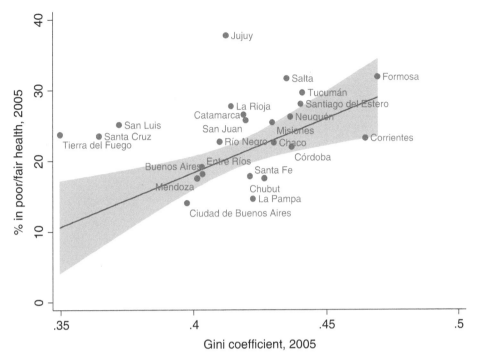

Figure 1. Scatterplot of 2005 income distribution and 2005 self-rated health by province ($r = 0.58$, $p < 0.01$).
Note: Shaded areas in both scatterplots represent 95% confidence intervals.

($\alpha = -1$), the association with poor health weakens and becomes non-significant ($r = 0.17$, $p = 0.42$).

The relationship between 2005 income inequality and 2009 health outcomes displays a similar pattern but with generally smaller correlation coefficients. The direction of the correlation between 2005 Gini and 2009 self-rated health remains

Table 2. Pearson correlation coefficients (r values) of provincial-level indicators of income inequality, poverty and self-rated health.

	Gini	GE(-1)	GE(0)	GE(1)	GE(2)	UBN	Poor health (2005)	Poor health (2009)
Gini	1.00							
GE(-1)	0.78***	1.00						
GE(0)	0.98***	0.88***	1.00					
GE(1)	0.98***	0.72***	0.95***	1.00				
GE(2)	0.90***	0.58***	0.85***	0.97***	1.00			
UBN	0.51*	0.28	0.47*	0.63***	0.74***	1.00		
Poor health (2005)	0.58**	0.17	0.48*	0.67***	0.75***	0.66***	1.00	
Poor health (2009)	0.37	0.03	0.29	0.51*	0.65***	0.81***	0.81***	1.00

*$p < 0.05$; **$p < 0.01$; ***$p < 0.001$, all two-tailed tests.

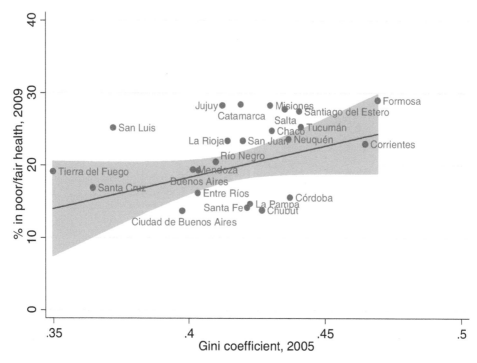

Figure 2. Scatterplot of 2005 income distribution and 2009 self-rated health by province ($r = 0.37$, $p = 0.07$).

positive ($r = 0.37$; see Figure 2), in line with the cross-sectional results, but this association does not attain statistical significance ($p = 0.07$).

Using the GE index, the gradient pattern observed previously remains in place, with the strongest correlation ($r = 0.65$, $p < 0.001$) again being detected using GE(2). The percentage of homes in a province with UBN was significantly associated with provincial Gini coefficients ($r = 0.51$, $p < 0.05$) and likewise displayed a gradient-like relationship with the GE index. The relationship between UBN and 2005/2009 health outcomes strengthens over the study period, with an increase in r from 0.66 to 0.81.

Discussion

These ecological analyses suggest that income inequality is associated with poor self-rated health in Argentina and that the strength of this association generally increases as the income inequality indicator becomes more and more sensitive to inequalities at the upper end of the distribution. This suggests that it is income gaps at the top of the income spectrum (i.e., among the rich) that may be ecologically associated with poorer levels of health. This pattern was observed in our cross-sectional analysis of 2005 data as well as in analyses that used health outcomes from 2009. This finding may be consistent with both the neo-material and psychosocial pathways (Kawachi et al. 1999, De Maio 2010). Increased income gaps at the top of the income distribution may signal a qualitatively different kind of inequality (Wen et al. 2003), a marked polarisation between the rich and the middle/poor classes. Fitting the rationale of the neo-material explanation, this polarisation may be associated with the deterioration of public infrastructure and the growth of gated communities and private community amenities. Qualitative research may be particularly useful in exploring this possibility. At the same time, increased income gaps at the top of the distribution may also be consistent with the psychosocial pathway, if the social comparisons that are critical to stress pathways are made between the poor/middle class and the rich (Buunk *et al.* 1997, Hagerty 2000, Pham-Kanter 2009).

When the 4-year time lag was introduced, the association between inequality and health generally weakened but the pattern remained consistent. The analysis therefore extends a relatively simple ecological analysis in two ways and finds that the extension by income inequality indicator generated new insight on a gradient-like effect with the income inequality indicator. The findings from the lagged analyses suggest that the health effects of income inequality may be more temporally limited than previously theorised, with stronger correlations in cross-sectional analysis than in lagged analysis. Future studies should examine this effect using a longer follow-up period.

When the income inequality indicator was sensitive to inequalities at the bottom of the distribution ($GE(-1)$), the association between inequality and poor health failed to reach statistical significance and the value of the correlation coefficient approached 0 (decreasing from $r = 0.17$ in 2005 to $r = 0.03$ in 2009). This suggests that theories of the health effects of income inequality need to be attuned to qualitative differences in inequalities; inequalities at the bottom of the income spectrum – despite mathematically contributing to a Gini coefficient – can actually signal pro-poor economic effects that improve the living conditions of the poor (Wen *et al.* 2003) or at the very least attenuate underlying health effects of income inequality. In other words, because Lorenz curves can intersect and qualitatively different distributions may therefore yield similar Gini coefficients, it is important to operationalise income inequality with a range of indicators – the Gini coefficient is known to be sensitive to inequalities in the middle of the spectrum and the GE index offers a sensitivity parameter that allows researchers to examine gradient effects.

Until now, the conventional practice in this area of research has been to treat the choice of income inequality indicator as a methodological nuisance – alternative measures are generally used only to support the choice of the Gini coefficient, and little, if any, attention has been given to the interpretation of how alternative measures may be correlated with health outcomes. However, instead of being a methodological nuisance, the use of a range of inequality indicators, such as those offered by the GE index, in studies such as these may be the source of new insight on how income distribution functions as a social determinant of health. These results indicate that it is increasing income gaps at the top end of the distribution that is particularly associated with poor population health.

There are three important limitations to this analysis. The first is the reliance on self-rated health and income data. A large segment of the income inequality – health literature has relied on self-rated health status (Lynch *et al.* 2004, Wilkinson and Pickett 2006, 2007), as it has been found to be highly predictive of actual health status, including subsequent morbidity (Kennedy *et al.* 1998) and mortality (Idler and Benyamini 1997, Blakely *et al.* 2002). At the same time, some studies have raised questions regarding the validity (Sen 2002, De Maio 2007a) and reliability (Crossley and Kennedy 2002) of self-rated health questions; however, self-rated health remains an accepted and widely used measure in the income inequality literature and in the

Southern Cone countries of Latin America. Future analysis should examine the robustness of these conclusions by using other indicators of provincial-level health status, including cause-specific mortality data as well as risk factor data that the ENFR was specifically designed to collect. In the absence of tax-based register data, we have relied on ENFR questions of self-reported income. As is the case with self-reported health, self-reported income is liable to measurement error. In particular, we may expect an under-reporting of income among higher income groups. Previous research from Argentina suggests that this may be a problem (Javier *et al.* 1995, Gasparini and Escudero 2001), and this could result in artificially low indicators of inequality. At the same time, error can also be expected in the income reporting of individuals involved in the informal economy. This may lead to an underestimate of the income of the poor and lower middle class. Future analyses could build on this work by considering measures of wealth inequality, along with measures of income inequality.

A second limitation is the reliance on aggregate-level analysis. Limitations of this type of analysis, including problems of ecological fallacy (Robinson 1950, Schwartz 1994, Pearce 2000) and the associated inability to distinguish contextual from compositional effects (Diez-Roux 2002), are well known, and the conclusions we can draw from these analyses are as a consequence limited. In addition, correlation analyses offer a very limited capacity for establishing cause–effect relationships, particularly if it is not possible to adjust for potential co-founders due to a relatively low number of ecological units, as is the case with Argentine provinces. Exploratory analyses utilising ordinary least squares (OLS) regression suggest that the Gini coefficient's effect may not be robust to the inclusion of UBN as an additional covariate, whereas the GE(2) unadjusted result is indeed stable and remains significant with the inclusion of provincial UBN (regression coefficients of 0.58, $p < 0.001$ in the unadjusted model and 0.44, $p < 0.05$ in the adjusted model; in both cases, GE(2) was centred around its mean). However, as we have only 24 ecological units, the validity of analysing these data with multiple regressions is questionable.

Given the existing theoretical work on pathways linking income inequality to health, the strength of these analyses does not rest on an ability to test specific causal pathways but for exploring the robustness of the hypothesis to changes in methodology. Indeed, our correlations may be confounded by region-specific fixed effects that are not accounted for in these exploratory analyses. Despite this limitation, ecological correlations remain a key building block in empirical research on the health effects of income inequality. Furthermore, given on-going debates in the literature over the appropriateness of multi-level strategies that control for individual-level income (Wilkinson and Pickett 2009a, Bernburg 2010), aggregate-level studies remain an important branch of the field.

Another limitation is rooted in the availability of data sources; as of now, only two waves of the ENFR have been carried out and this restricted our analysis to a 4-year lag. Our results may therefore be specific to Argentina's experiences in the period 2005–2009; a period of economic recovery from the devastating crisis of 2001–2003 (Rock 2002, Lloyd-Sherlock 2005). If more waves of the ENFR are implemented, longer lag effects can be tested. Given existing work that suggests that lags of 10–15 years are appropriate (Blakely *et al.* 2000, Leigh and Jencks 2007), this is a particularly important issue for future studies to investigate. Longer follow-up periods may be associated with increased variation of both income inequality and health, thereby increasing the statistical power of the analysis (Blakely 2000). This will be of help to better map out the dynamics of the health effects of income inequality. Longer periods of study are also needed for the 'historically deep' analysis that is required to fully test the complex theoretical ideas underlying the income inequality model; this calls for a truly interdisciplinary lens, blending social epidemiology, sociology and political economy (Coburn 2000, 2004).

Future studies should seek to identify potential heterogeneity in the estimated relationship between inequality and health. For example, a gender-based analysis could seek to map out differential effects of income inequality on men and women. Studies are also needed to situate the health effects of income inequality in Argentina in a regional context, perhaps through cross-national comparisons with the neighbouring Southern Cone countries. Such work may identify 'natural experiments', which may add particular insight to our understanding of how social and political processes related to inequality influence population health. Cross-national analysis also offers greater potential for multilevel techniques, as the number of ecological would increase.

Despite a large and growing scholarly literature, a consensus on the income inequality–population health hypothesis has not been reached. The policy implications of this body of work are contested (Starfield and Birn 2007). Much remains to be done on methodological and theoretical levels, yet the results of this study point towards the need for more consideration on how the choice of income inequality indicator may influence results. A renewed appreciation of the sensitivity of the hypothesis to the choice of the inequality indicator as well as an awareness of the temporal dynamics of the effect may yield valuable insight and, in the process, contribute to new understanding of how income redistribution may be means by which to improve population health.

Acknowledgements

Funding from the Social Sciences and Humanities Research Council of Canada (SSHRC) is gratefully acknowledged (De Maio).

References

Atkinson, A.B., 1975. *The economics of inequality*. Oxford: Claredon Press.

Auger, N., Giraud, J., and Daniel, M., 2009. The joint in uence of area income, income inequality, and immigrant density on adverse birth outcomes: a population-based study. *BioMed Central Public Health*, 9, 237.

Bernburg, J.G., 2010. Relative deprivation theory does not imply a contextual effect of country-level inequality on poor health. A commentary on Jen, Jones, and Johnston (68:4, 2009). *Social Science and Medicine*, 70 (4), 493–495; discussion 498–500.

Blakely, T., Kennedy, B.P., Glass, R., and Kawachi, I., 2000. What is the lag time between income inequality and health status? *Journal of Epidemiology and Community Health*, 54 (4), 318–319.

Blakely, T., Lochner, K., and Kawachi, I., 2002. Metropolitan area income inequality and self-rated health – a multilevel study. *Social Science and Medicine*, 54, 65–77.

Böckerman, P., Johansson, E., Helakorpi, S., and Uutela, A., 2009. Economic inequality and population health: looking beyond aggregate indicators. *Sociology of Health and Illness*, 31 (3), 422–440.

Breckenkamp, J., Mielck, A., and Razum, O., 2007. Health inequalities in Germany: do regional-level variables explain differentials in cardiovascular risk? *BioMed Central Public Health*, 7, 132.

Brunner, E., 1997. Stress and the biology of inequality. *British Medical Journal*, 314 (7092), 1472–1476.

Buunk, B.P., Gibbons, F.X., and Reis-Bergan, M., 1997. Social comparison in health and illness: a historical overview. *In*: B.P. Buunk and F.X. Gibbons, eds. *Health, coping, and well-being: perspectives from social comparison theory*. London: LEA, 1–24.

Cavalini, L.T. and De Leon, A.C., 2008. Morbidity and mortality in Brazilian municipalities: a multilevel study of the association between socioeconomic and healthcare indicators. *International Journal of Epidemiology*, 37 (4), 775–783.

Chakravarty, S.R., 2009. *Inequality, polarization and poverty: advances in distributional analysis*. New York: Springer.

Coburn, D., 2000. Income inequality, social cohesion and the health status of populations: the role of neo-liberalism. *Social Science and Medicine*, 51 (1), 135–146.

Coburn, D., 2004. Beyond the income inequality hypothesis: class, neo-liberalism, and health inequalities. *Social Science and Medicine*, 58 (1), 41–56.

Cowell, F.A., 1995. *Measuring inequality*. 2nd ed. London: Prentice Hall.

Crossley, T.F. and Kennedy, S., 2002. The reliability of self-assessed health status. *Journal of Health Economics*, 21, 643–658.

De Maio, F.G., 2007a. Health inequalities in Argentina: patterns, contradictions and implications. *Health Sociology Review*, 16 (3–4), 279–291.

De Maio, F.G., 2007b. Income inequality measures. *Journal of Epidemiology and Community Health*, 61 (10), 849–852.

De Maio, F.G., 2008. Ecological analysis of the health effects of income inequality in Argentina. *Public Health*, 122 (5), 487–496.

De Maio, F.G., 2010. *Health and social theory*. Basingstoke, UK: Palgrave Macmillan.

De Maio, F.G., 2012. Advancing the income inequality – health hypothesis. *Critical Public Health*, 22 (1), 39–46.

De Maio, F.G., Linetzky, B., and Virgolini, M., 2009. An average/deprivation/inequality (ADI) analysis of chronic disease outcomes and risk factors in Argentina. *Population Health Metrics*, 7, 8.

De Vaus, D., 2002. *Surveys in social research*. St. Leonards, Australia: Routledge.

De Vogli, R., Mistry, R., Gnesotto, R., and Cornia, G.A., 2005. Has the relation between income inequality and life expectancy disappeared? Evidence from Italy and top industrialised countries. *Journal of Epidemiology and Community Health*, 59 (2), 158–162.

Diez-Roux, A.V., 2002. A glossary for multilevel analysis. *Journal of Epidemiology and Community Health*, 56 (8), 588–594.

Dunn, J.R., Schaub, P., and Ross, N.A., 2007. Unpacking income inequality and population health: the peculiar absence of geography. *Canadian Journal of Public Health*, 98 (Suppl. 1), S10–S17.

Ellison, G.T.H., 2002. Letting the Gini out of the bottle? Challenges facing the relative income hypothesis. *Social Science and Medicine*, 54 (4), 561–576.

Ferrante, D., 2006. Mortalidad por enfermedades crónicas: Demasiado tarde para lágrimas. *Revista Argentina de Cardiologia*, 74 (3), 196–197.

Ferrante, D. and Virgolini, M., 2007. Encuesta Nacional de Factores de Riesgo 2005: Resultados principales. *Revista Argentina de Cardiologia*, 75, 20–29.

Fleischer, N.L., Diez Roux, A.V., Alazraqui, M., and Spinelli, H., 2008. Social patterning of chronic disease risk factors in a Latin American city. *Journal of Urban Health*, 85 (6), 923–937.

Gasparini, L. and Escudero, W.S., 2001. Assessing aggregate welfare: growth and inequality in Argentina. *Cuadernos de Economía*, 38 (113), 49–71.

Hagerty, M.R., 2000. Social comparisons of income in one's community: evidence from national surveys of income and happiness. *Journal of Personality and Social Psychology*, 78 (4), 764–771.

Hey, J.D. and Lambert, P.J., 1980. Relative deprivation and the Gini coefficient: comment. *Quarterly Journal of Economics*, 95 (3), 567–573.

Idler, E.L. and Benyamini, Y., 1997. Self-rated health and mortality: a review of twenty-seven community studies. *Journal of Health and Social Behavior*, 38 (1), 21–37.

INDEC, 2003. Aquí se cuenta. *Revista Informativa del Censo 2001*, (7), 1–6. Available from: http://www.indec.gov.ar/webcenso/aquisecuenta/Aqui7.pdf

Javier, E., Lee, H., and Leipziger, D., 1995. *Argentina's poor: a profile*. Washington, DC: World Bank. (Report No. 13318-AR)

Jenkins, S.P., 1991. The measurement of income inequality. *In*: L. Osberg, ed. *Economic inequality and poverty: international perspectives*. London: M.E. Sharpe, 3–38.

Jenkins, S.P., 1999. Analysis of income distributions. *Stata Technical Bulletin*, 48, 4–18.

Kahn, R.S., Wise, P.H., Kennedy, B.P., and Kawachi, I., 2000. State income inequality, household income, and maternal mental and physical health: cross sectional national survey. *British Medical Journal*, 321 (7272), 1311–1315.

Kawachi, I. and Kennedy, B.P., 1997. The relationship of income inequality to mortality: does the choice of indicator matter? *Social Science and Medicine*, 45 (7), 1121–1127.

Kawachi, I., Kennedy, B.P., and Wilkinson, R.G., 1999. *The society and population health reader: income inequality and health*. New York: The New Press.

Kennedy, B.P., Kawachi, I., Glass, R., and Prothrow-Stith, D., 1998. Income distribution, socioeconomic status, and self rated health in the United States: multilevel analysis. *British Medical Journal*, 317 (7163), 917–921.

Laporte, A. and Ferguson, B.S., 2003. Income inequality and mortality: time series evidence from Canada. *Health Policy*, 66 (1), 107–117.

Leigh, A. and Jencks, C., 2007. Inequality and mortality: long-run evidence from a panel of countries. *Journal of Health Economics*, 26 (1), 1–24.

Lloyd-Sherlock, P., 2005. Health sector reform in Argentina: a cautionary tale. *Social Science and Medicine*, 60 (8), 1893–1903.

Lynch, J., Davey Smith, G., Harper, S., Hillermeier, M., Ross, N., Kaplan, G.A., and Wolfson, M., 2004. Is income inequality a determinant of population health? Part 1. A systematic review. *The Milbank Quarterly*, 82 (1), 5–99.

Lynch, J., Harper, S., and Davey Smith, G., 2003. Plugging leaks and repelling boarders – where to next for the SS income inequality? *International Journal of Epidemiology*, 32 (6), 1029–1036.

Lynch, J., Harper, S., Kaplan, G.A., and Davey Smith, G., 2005. Associations between income inequality and mortality among US states: the importance of time period and source of income data. *American Journal of Public Health*, 95 (8), 1424–1430.

Marín, G.H., Rivadulla, P., Negro, L., Gelemur, M., Etchegoyen, G., and GIS, 2008. Estudio poblacional de prevalencia de anemia en población adulta de Buenos Aires, Argentina. *Atención Primaria*, 40 (3), 133–138.

Mcewen, B.S., 1998. Protective and damaging effects of stress mediators. *New England Journal of Medicine*, 338 (3), 171–179.

Montilva, M., Ferrer, M.A., Nieto, R., Yudith, O., Durán, L., and Mendoza, M.A., 2003. Uso del método Necesidades Básicas Insatisfechas en la detección de comunidades con riesgo de desnutrición. *Anales Venezolanos de Nutrición*, 16 (1), 16–22.

MSAL, 2011. *2ª Encuesta Nacional de Factores de Riesgo* [online]. Available from: http://www.msal.gov.ar/ENT/PDF/ENFR_2009_presentacion%20ppt.pdf [Accessed 4 February 2011].

Osler, M., Christensen, U., Due, P., Lund, R., Andersen, I., Diderichsen, F., and Prescott, E., 2003. Income inequality and ischaemic heart disease in Danish men and women. *International Journal of Epidemiology*, 32 (3), 375–380.

Osler, M., Prescott, E., Gronbaek, M., Christensen, U., Due, P., and Engholm, G., 2002. Income inequality, individual income, and mortality in Danish adults: analysis of pooled data from two cohort studies. *British Medical Journal*, 324 (7328), 13.

Pearce, N., 2000. The ecological fallacy strikes back. *Journal of Epidemiology and Community Health*, 54 (5), 326–327.

Pei, X. and Rodriguez, E., 2006. Provincial income inequality and self-reported health status in China during 1991-7. *Journal of Epidemiology and Community Health*, 60 (12), 1065–1069.

Peña, R., Wall, S., and Persson, L.A., 2000. The effect of poverty, social inequity, and maternal education on infant mortality in Nicaragua, 1988-1993. *American Journal of Public Health*, 90 (1), 64–69.

Pham-Kanter, G., 2009. Social comparisons and health: can having richer friends and neighbors make you sick? *Social Science and Medicine*, 69 (3), 335–344.

Robinson, W.S., 1950. Ecological correlations and the behavior of individuals. *American Sociological Review*, 15, 351–357.

Rock, D., 2002. Racking Argentina. *New Left Review*, 17, 55–86.

Ross, N.A., Wolfson, M.C., Dunn, J.R., Berthelot, J.M., Kaplan, G.A., and Lynch, J.W., 2000. Relation between income inequality and mortality in Canada and in the United States: cross sectional assessment using census data and vital statistics. *British Medical Journal*, 320 (7239), 898–902.

Schwartz, S., 1994. The fallacy of the ecological fallacy: the potential misuse of a concept and the consequences. *American Journal of Public Health*, 84 (5), 819–824.

Sen, A., 2002. Health: perception versus observation. *British Medical Journal*, 324 (7342), 860–861.

Shibuya, K., Hashimoto, H., and Yano, E., 2002. Individual income, income distribution, and self rated health in Japan: cross sectional analysis of nationally representative sample. *British Medical Journal*, 324 (7328), 16.

Starfield, B. and Birn, A.E., 2007. Income redistribution is not enough: income inequality, social welfare programs, and achieving equity in health. *Journal of Epidemiology and Community Health*, 61 (12), 1038–1041.

Subramanian, S.V., Delgado, I., Jadue, L., Vega, J., and Kawachi, I., 2003. Income inequality and health: multilevel analysis of Chilean communities. *Journal of Epidemiology and Community Health*, 57 (11), 844–848.

Subramanian, S.V. and Kawachi, I., 2003. In defence of the income inequality hypothesis. *International Journal of Epidemiology*, 32, 1037–1040.

Veenstra, G., 2002. Income inequality and health. Coastal communities in British Columbia, Canada. *Canadian Journal of Public Health*, 93 (5), 374–379.

Weich, S., Lewis, G., and Jenkins, S.P., 2002. Income inequality and self rated health in Britain. *Journal of Epidemiology and Community Health*, 56 (6), 436–441.

Wen, M., Browning, C.R., and Cagney, K.A., 2003. Poverty, af uence, and income inequality: neighborhood economic structure and its implications for health. *Social Science and Medicine*, 57 (5), 843–860.

Wilkinson, R.G., 2000. *Mind the gap: hierarchies, health and human evolution*. London: Weidenfeld and Nicolson.

Wilkinson, R.G. and Pickett, K.E., 2006. Income inequality and population health: a review and explanation of the evidence. *Social Science and Medicine*, 62 (7), 1768–1784.

Wilkinson, R.G. and Pickett, K.E., 2007. The problems of relative deprivation: why some societies do better than others. *Social Science and Medicine*, 65 (9), 1965–1978.

Wilkinson, R.G. and Pickett, K.E., 2008. Income inequality and socioeconomic gradients in mortality. *American Journal of Public Health*, 98 (4), 699–704.

Wilkinson, R.G. and Pickett, K.E., 2009a. Income inequality and social dysfunciton. *Annual Review of Sociology*, 35, 493–511.

Wilkinson, R.G. and Pickett, K.E., 2009b. *The spirit level: why more equal societies almost always do better*. London: Allen Lane.

Index

Adolescent Reproductive Health Program 27, 28
advocacy organizations 104
affirmative action policies 64
Almeida Filho, Naomar de 76–82
Andean culture 37–8, 43–4; *see also* Bolivian
  migrant women
Argentina: cancer control in 5–17; Chagas
  disease (CD) in 3, 90–1; community
  participation and Chagas disease in 89–100;
  Encuesta Permanente de Hogares (EPH)
  115; and frontline practitioners' priorities
  for cancer patients' care 9–16; health care
  services of 12–14; Ministry of Health 114;
  non-communicable diseases in 113; political
  influence and cancer treatment 14; social
  treatment of cancer study 8; and South
  American migrants 37
Argentine National Risk Factor Surveys
  112–21

Barreto, Maurício 76, 78
Bolivian migrant women: and culture 42;
  interviews 38–44; reproductive health 35–45;
  and self-care 41
Brazil: Bahia in 65; inequalities in 64, 67; military
  dictatorship in 61; Ministry of Health 65;
  political crisis in 62; racial issue in 67; social
  disparities producing health inequities and
  shaping sickle cell disorder in 61–70; system of
  racial classification in 67
Brazilian Constitution 62
Brazilian Institute of Geography and Statistics
  (IBGE) 64
Brazilian National Health System (SUS) 62, 64
Brazilian Universal Health System 69
British Household Panel Survey 114
bureaucratic mechanisms: and radiology services
  12–13; and social insurance 12

Canadian Institutes for Health Research 108
cancer: control in Argentina 5–17; and Latin
  America 7; overview 5; and socio-economic
  status 6; treatment and political influence 14

cancer patients: and health services' staffs 9–16;
  and personal voluntarism 14–16; social and
  cultural characteristics of 11–12
*Centro Nacional para la Equidad de Género y
  la Salud Reproductiva* (National Centre for
  Gender Equity and Reproductive Health) 24
Chagas disease (CD) 89–100, 105–6; in
  Argentina 3, 90–1; community participation in
  surveillance and disease control 91–2; globalist
  perspective on 108; in non-endemic countries
  103–8; spectre of a 'globalized' chagas 106–8
collective health 74–5; defined 75; modern
  epidemiology and 76
Collective Health 76
Connell, Raewyn 1, 4n1
contraceptive methods 25, 26
'cultural epidemiology' 2, 74, 75, 79–84
culture: and Bolivian migrant women 42–3;
  and self-care 42–3

Declaration of Alma Ata 91
Diez Roux, Ana 76
direct racism 62; *see also* racism
doctor–patient relationships (DPR): described 47;
  and eHealth 49, 51–3; facilitators of 56; health
  communication 48; models 51, 54; obstacles
  of 56; overview 47–8; patient satisfaction 50;
  process of transformation in 55; technological
  changes to 49; thematisation of 49

eHealth 49, 51–3, 54; described 51–2; limitation
  of 55; and use of internet 52
*Encuesta Nacional de la Dinámica Demográfica-
  ENADID* (National Demographic Dynamics
  Survey-NDDS) 30
Encuesta Permanente de Hogares (EPH) 115
epidemiology: cultural 79; intercultural 83;
  modern 75–8; social 82; sociocultural 81–2
'Epidemiology without numbers' (Almeida
  Filho) 76
'ethnoepidemiology' 79–81
'ethnoracial hierarchy' 61
'Even Start in Life' 23

125

San Quintín area *see* northwestern Mexico
schistosomiasis 108
Science 75
self-care: and Bolivian migrant women 41; and
   culture 42–3
sexual health: of indigenous migrant women in
   northwestern Mexico 20–33; and international
   organisations 22; World Health Organization
   on 23
sexuality: cultural beliefs on 32; indigenous
   migrant women on 25–6
sexually transmitted diseases 27
sexual rights, and indigenous migrant women 29
'sick immigrant' phobia 103–8
sickle cell disorder (SCD): as 'childhood disease'
   63; from a global scenario to the local context
   of Brazil 63–6; racism taken as a form of social
   inequity affecting 66–9; social disparities and
   61–70
social and health inequities 89–100
social disparities: health inequities and 61–70;
   sickle cell disorder and 61–70
social epidemiology 82
social insurance, and bureaucratic
   mechanisms 12
social medicine 1, 2, 75, 78

sociocultural epidemiology 81–2
socio/ethno-epidemiologies: criticisms of
   modern epidemiology 75–8; one or many 78–9
sociology of health literature, and Latin
   America 1–3
Southern Theory (Connell) 1
Swidler, Ann 42

Triatoma infestans 92
Triatoma pallidipennis 99
Trypanosoma cruzi (T. cruzi) 90–1, 105–7

United Nations 22
US National Institutes of Health 108

vinchucas 89–99

Weiss, Mitchell G. 79
women: on information about sexuality 25–6;
   jornaleras in Mexico 21; *see also specific
   entries*
World Conference on Social Development 22
World Health Organization (WHO) 69, 90,
   103–4; Commission on Social Determinants of
   Health (CSDH) 77; on reproductive health 23;
   on sexual health 23

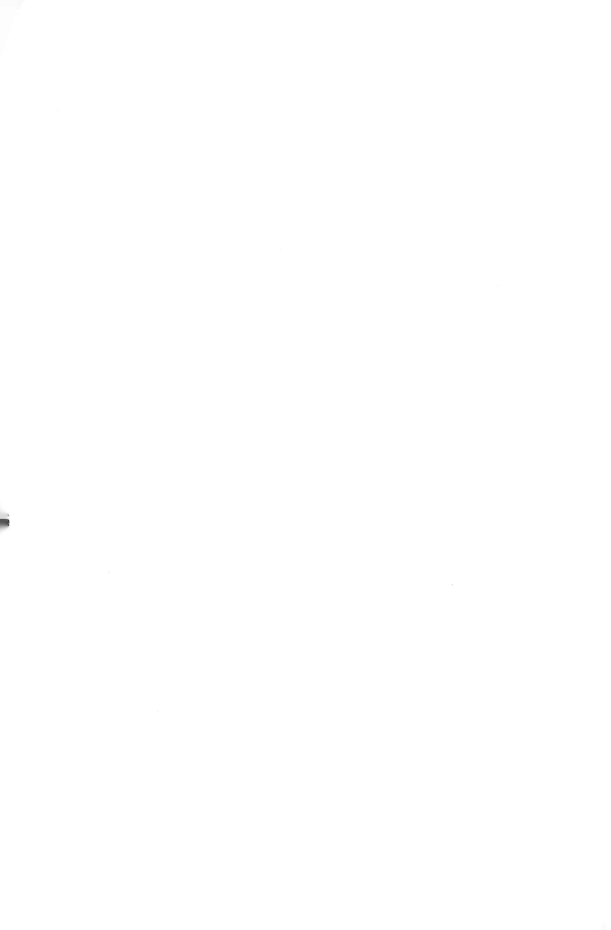

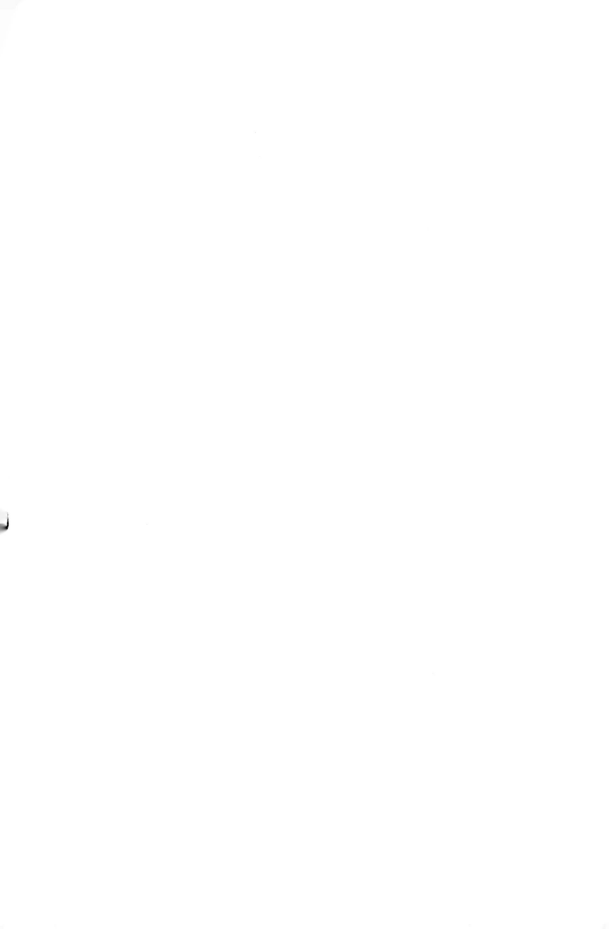